I0838785

Alternative and Complementary Therapies for Rheumatoid Arthritis

Alternative and Complementary Therapies for Rheumatoid Arthritis

Victor Asher

Other Books by Victor Asher

Dedication

This book is dedicated to God for His grace and wisdom, to my family, to my beautiful readers who will find this book relevant to them, and to everyone who has loved, supported, and encouraged me along the way. I would not be in the position I am in today without your unshakable faith in me. I dedicate this book to all my readers especially those with rheumatoid arthritis and pray this to be of help to you all.

Table of Contents

Acknowledgement

I want to sincerely thank God for providing the means and insight that guided me during the writing of this book. I cannot forget my family members, whose encouragement and support have given me bravery and motivation throughout the process.

Thank you to my editor and publisher for their crucial advice and help in bringing this project to its successful conclusion. I would like to express my gratitude to everyone who so kindly contributed their time and knowledge to this project and added their wisdom. I want to express my gratitude to my friends as well, I appreciate all of your steadfast love and support throughout the journey.

Finally, I extend my thanks to each and every one of you for purchasing and reading my work. I am thankful it met your needs and added to your knowledge. I sincerely value each and every one of you and think you're all fantastic.

Introduction

Rheumatoid arthritis (RA) is a chronic autoimmune disease that affects millions of people worldwide, causing pain, inflammation, and joint damage. Living with rheumatoid arthritis (RA) can be a challenging journey, as the chronic pain, inflammation, and joint stiffness often disrupt daily life. While conventional medical treatments play a vital role in managing RA, many individuals seek additional avenues to alleviate symptoms, improve quality of life, and regain control over their health. This is where alternative and complementary therapies come into the picture.

"Alternative and Complementary Therapies for Rheumatoid Arthritis" offers a comprehensive exploration of these non-traditional approaches to RA management. This book is designed to empower individuals with RA, their loved ones, and healthcare professionals with the knowledge and understanding of alternative options that can complement conventional treatments and improve overall well-being.

In this book, we will delve into a wide range of alternative and complementary therapies, each offering unique benefits for those living with RA. From ancient practices like acupuncture and massage therapy to mind-body techniques such as meditation and yoga, we uncover the power of these therapies in alleviating pain, reducing inflammation, and enhancing physical and emotional well-being.

Evidence-based research forms the foundation of our exploration, ensuring that the information provided is grounded in scientific understanding and practical application. We delve into the mechanisms behind each therapy, examining how they interact with the body and the potential benefits they offer specifically for RA symptoms.

Safety and effectiveness are paramount considerations in any approach to managing RA. Throughout this book, we discuss factors to consider when integrating alternative and complementary therapies into your treatment plan. We provide guidance on finding qualified practitioners, navigating potential interactions with medications, and ensuring that your choices align with your unique needs and circumstances.

This book goes beyond mere information, as it aims to empower individuals with RA to take an active role in their own well-being. We provide practical tips, strategies, and guidance on how to incorporate these therapies into daily life. Whether you are exploring acupuncture, considering massage therapy, or seeking solace in mind-body practices, this book serves as your comprehensive roadmap, assisting you in making informed decisions and finding the right path towards relief and resilience.

Ultimately, "Alternative and Complementary Therapies for Rheumatoid Arthritis" serves as a beacon of hope, guiding you towards a holistic and integrated approach to managing RA. By embracing these alternative options alongside conventional treatments, you can uncover new avenues for pain relief, increased mobility, and overall improved quality of life. Together, let us embark on this journey of exploration, empowerment, and healing.

Chapter 1

Understanding Alternative and Complementary Therapies for Rheumatoid Arthritis

Alternative and complementary therapies for rheumatoid arthritis refer to non-traditional approaches that individuals with RA may explore alongside or in conjunction with conventional medical treatments. These therapies aim to provide additional relief, support, and improvement in managing the symptoms and overall well-being of individuals living with rheumatoid arthritis.

"Alternative" therapies are those that are used in place of conventional medical treatments. They may include practices rooted in ancient traditions, such as acupuncture, herbal remedies, or mind-body techniques like meditation and yoga. Alternative therapies offer alternative pathways to address the challenges associated with RA, often focusing on holistic approaches and natural healing methods.

"Complementary" therapies, on the other hand, are used alongside conventional medical treatments. They complement the existing treatment plan and aim to enhance its effectiveness or provide additional benefits. Complementary therapies may include massage therapy, hydrotherapy, heat and cold therapy, and dietary supplements. These therapies are meant to work in synergy with conventional treatments, offering a comprehensive and integrated approach to managing RA.

The purpose of alternative and complementary therapies for rheumatoid arthritis is to empower individuals with RA to take an active role in their own health and well-being. These therapies often focus on promoting physical and emotional balance, reducing pain and inflammation, improving mobility, and enhancing overall quality of life. While they may not replace conventional treatments, they provide individuals with additional options to explore, tailored to their unique needs and preferences.

It is important to note that when considering alternative and complementary therapies, individuals should consult with their healthcare providers. This ensures a collaborative and informed approach, considering potential interactions with medications, safety considerations, and overall integration with the existing treatment plan. By embracing alternative and complementary therapies alongside conventional treatments, individuals with RA can access a broader range of options to optimize their management and enhance their overall well-being.

Alternative Therapy

Alternative therapy refers to non-conventional or non-mainstream approaches to healthcare and healing that are used in place of or alongside conventional medical treatments. These therapies often emphasize a holistic and integrative approach, addressing the physical, emotional, and spiritual aspects of an individual's well-being.

Alternative therapies encompass a wide range of practices, including but not limited to:

1. Acupuncture

A traditional Chinese therapy that involves the insertion of thin needles into specific points on the body to stimulate energy flow and promote healing.

2. Herbal Medicine

The use of plants, herbs, and botanical extracts to treat various health conditions and promote overall well-being.

3. Homeopathy

A system of medicine based on the principle of "like cures like," where highly diluted substances are used to stimulate the body's self-healing abilities.

4. Naturopathy

An approach that emphasizes natural remedies, such as nutrition, herbal medicine, and lifestyle modifications, to support the body's inherent healing capacity.

5. Ayurveda

A traditional Indian system of medicine that focuses on balancing the body, mind, and spirit through practices like herbal remedies, diet, yoga, and meditation.

6. Energy Healing

Therapies that work with the body's energy fields, such as Reiki or Qigong, to promote relaxation, balance, and well-being.

7. Chiropractic Care

A hands-on approach that focuses on the alignment of the spine and musculoskeletal system to improve overall health and alleviate pain.

8. Mind-Body Practices

Techniques like meditation, yoga, tai chi, and guided imagery that promote relaxation, stress reduction, and mind-body connection.

It's important to note that while alternative therapies can offer potential benefits, their effectiveness and safety may vary, and scientific evidence supporting their use may be limited. It is advisable to consult with healthcare professionals and ensure open communication to integrate alternative therapies safely and effectively into a comprehensive healthcare plan. Additionally, it is essential to inform healthcare providers about any alternative therapies being used to prevent potential interactions or contraindications with conventional treatments.

Complementary Therapies

Complementary therapies are non-conventional approaches to healthcare that are used alongside or in conjunction with conventional medical treatments. These therapies are intended to complement and enhance the effectiveness of traditional medical interventions, providing additional support and promoting overall well-being.

Complementary therapies take into account the physical, emotional, and spiritual aspects of an individual's health, aiming to optimize the body's natural healing abilities and improve quality of life. They are often used in conjunction with conventional treatments to address symptoms, manage side effects, reduce stress, and promote a sense of balance and well-being.

Examples of complementary therapies include:

1. Massage Therapy

The manipulation of soft tissues through various techniques, such as Swedish massage or deep tissue massage, to relieve muscle tension, reduce pain, and promote relaxation.

2. Yoga

An ancient practice that combines physical postures, breathing exercises, and meditation to improve flexibility, strength, balance, and mental clarity.

3. Meditation

A technique that involves focusing the mind and cultivating a state of calm and mindfulness, which can reduce stress, anxiety, and promote emotional well-being.

4. Mindfulness-Based Stress Reduction (MBSR)

A program that combines mindfulness meditation, gentle movement, and cognitive-behavioral techniques to help individuals manage stress, pain, and enhance overall well-being.

5. Art Therapy

The use of creative expression through art, such as painting, drawing, or sculpting, to facilitate emotional healing, self-exploration, and stress reduction.

6. Music Therapy

The use of music and sound to promote relaxation, reduce pain, and enhance emotional well-being.

7. Tai Chi

A gentle martial art form that combines slow, flowing movements, deep breathing, and meditation, promoting balance, flexibility, and stress reduction.

8. Dietary Supplements

The use of specific vitamins, minerals, or herbal remedies as supplements to support overall health and address specific deficiencies or health concerns.

Complementary therapies can provide individuals with additional tools to manage their health and well-being, offering a holistic approach that complements traditional medical treatments. It is important to discuss the use of complementary therapies with healthcare professionals to ensure safe and effective integration, as well as to maintain open communication about any potential interactions or contraindications with conventional treatments.

Exploring the Role of Alternative and Complementary Therapies

Alternative and complementary therapies play a significant role in the management of rheumatoid arthritis (RA) by providing additional avenues for symptom relief, improving overall well-being, and empowering individuals in their journey with this chronic condition. While conventional medical treatments remain the primary approach, alternative and complementary therapies offer complementary benefits that can enhance the effectiveness of conventional treatments and provide a more holistic approach to RA management.

The roles include:

1. Symptom Relief

Many alternative and complementary therapies aim to alleviate pain, reduce inflammation, and improve joint mobility. Therapies such as acupuncture, massage therapy, and heat/cold therapy can provide targeted relief for specific areas of pain and discomfort. Herbal remedies and dietary supplements may also offer anti-inflammatory properties that help manage RA symptoms.

2. Emotional Well-being

Living with RA can take a toll on mental and emotional health. Alternative therapies such as meditation, yoga, and mindfulness practices can reduce stress, anxiety, and depression associated with RA. These practices promote relaxation, improve mood, and enhance overall emotional well-being, which can positively impact the management of RA.

3. Physical Function and Mobility

Complementary therapies like yoga, tai chi, and gentle exercise programs can improve strength, flexibility, and joint range of motion. These activities help manage pain, prevent muscle atrophy, and maintain overall physical function and mobility, enhancing the ability to perform daily activities and reducing the impact of RA on quality of life.

4. Self-Empowerment and Active Participation

Alternative and complementary therapies often emphasize self-care, self-management, and active participation in the healing process. Engaging in therapies like meditation, guided imagery, or art therapy allows individuals to take an active role in their own well-being, fostering a sense of empowerment, control, and resilience in managing RA.

5. Quality of Life Improvement

The holistic approach of alternative and complementary therapies addresses not only physical symptoms but also the emotional, social, and spiritual aspects of well-being. By incorporating these therapies into a comprehensive treatment plan, individuals with RA can experience an overall improvement in their quality of life, including better sleep, increased energy levels, improved mood, and a greater sense of well-being.

It is important to note that alternative and complementary therapies should be used alongside conventional medical treatments and in consultation with healthcare professionals. Open communication with healthcare providers ensures proper coordination and integration of therapies, consideration of potential interactions or contraindications, and monitoring of overall health and progress.

By embracing alternative and complementary therapies as part of a holistic approach to RA management, individuals can expand their options, find relief, and actively participate in their own well-being, leading to a more comprehensive and personalized approach to living with rheumatoid arthritis.

Complementing Traditional Treatments: The Synergy of Conventional and Alternative Approaches

The integration of conventional and alternative approaches to healthcare is a topic that has gained significant attention in recent years. Complementing traditional treatments with alternative therapies can provide a holistic and comprehensive approach to healthcare, addressing not only the physical symptoms but also the mental, emotional, and spiritual well-being of individuals. This synergy between conventional and alternative approaches can offer a range of benefits to patients.

Conventional medicine, also known as allopathic or Western medicine, is based on scientific evidence, clinical trials, and rigorous research. It utilizes pharmaceutical drugs, surgeries, and other interventions to treat diseases and manage symptoms. Conventional medicine has made remarkable advancements in diagnosing and treating a wide range of health conditions and is particularly effective in acute and life-threatening situations.

However, conventional medicine may have limitations in certain areas, such as chronic disease management, pain management, and mental health. This is where alternative approaches can play a valuable role. Alternative medicine encompasses a diverse range of therapies, including acupuncture, herbal medicine, chiropractic care, naturopathy, homeopathy, and many others. These approaches often focus on supporting the body's natural healing processes and promoting overall well-being.

When conventional and alternative approaches are combined, they can provide a more comprehensive and patient-centered approach to healthcare.

Here are some ways in which the synergy between these two approaches can be beneficial:

1. Holistic Care

Alternative therapies often emphasize the connection between mind, body, and spirit. By incorporating these therapies alongside conventional treatments, patients can receive more holistic care that addresses their physical, emotional, and spiritual needs.

2. Personalized Treatment

Integrative medicine approaches consider each patient as an individual with unique needs. By combining conventional and alternative treatments, healthcare providers can tailor treatment plans to the specific needs and preferences of patients, enhancing the effectiveness of care.

3. Enhanced Symptom Management

Alternative therapies can provide additional tools for managing symptoms and side effects of conventional treatments. For example, cancer patients may use acupuncture to alleviate chemotherapy-induced nausea or practice meditation to reduce anxiety.

4. Prevention and Wellness Promotion

Alternative approaches often focus on preventive measures and lifestyle modifications to promote overall health and wellness. Integrating these strategies with conventional medicine can empower individuals to take an active role in their health and reduce the risk of developing chronic diseases.

5. Expanded Treatment Options

Some health conditions may not respond well to conventional treatments alone. In such cases, alternative therapies can offer additional treatment options, providing patients with more choices and potential avenues for healing.

It's important to note that the integration of conventional and alternative approaches should be done in a responsible and evidence-based manner. Collaboration and communication between healthcare providers from different disciplines are crucial to ensure patient safety and optimize outcomes.

In all, the synergy between conventional and alternative approaches to healthcare can offer numerous benefits to patients. By integrating these approaches, individuals can receive comprehensive care that addresses their physical, emotional, and spiritual well-being. This complementary approach has the potential to enhance treatment outcomes, improve symptom management, promote overall wellness, and empower individuals to take an active role in their health.

The Importance of an Integrative Approach to Rheumatoid Arthritis Management

Rheumatoid arthritis (RA) is a chronic autoimmune disease characterized by joint inflammation, pain, and progressive damage. The management of RA typically involves a combination of conventional medical treatments and lifestyle modifications. However, an emerging approach gaining recognition is the importance of an integrative approach to RA management.

1. Comprehensive Symptom Control

RA is a complex disease that affects multiple aspects of a person's health. Conventional medical treatments, such as disease-modifying antirheumatic drugs (DMARDs) and biologic agents, target the underlying inflammation and joint damage. However, integrating complementary therapies such as acupuncture, massage therapy, or herbal remedies can provide additional relief from pain, reduce inflammation, and improve overall joint function. By addressing multiple aspects of symptom control, an integrative approach can offer a more comprehensive strategy for managing RA symptoms.

2. Holistic Well-being

RA not only impacts the physical body but also affects emotional well-being, mental health, and overall quality of life. Integrating complementary therapies like mindfulness-based stress reduction, yoga, and meditation can help individuals cope with stress, reduce anxiety, and improve mental resilience. These practices promote a sense of relaxation, emotional balance, and overall well-being, complementing the conventional medical treatments and addressing the holistic needs of individuals with RA.

3. Empowerment and Active Participation

Adopting an integrative approach empowers individuals to take an active role in their RA management. Self-care practices, such as regular exercise, maintaining a balanced diet, and engaging in stress management techniques, allow individuals to actively contribute to their own well-being. This sense of empowerment fosters a greater sense of control and ownership over their condition, leading to increased motivation and adherence to treatment plans.

4. Personalized Treatment Plans

Each individual with RA has unique needs, preferences, and responses to different treatment modalities. An integrative approach recognizes the importance of tailoring treatment plans to meet individual requirements. Collaborating with healthcare providers who specialize in integrative medicine allows for the development of personalized treatment plans that incorporate a combination of conventional and complementary therapies. This personalized approach considers the individual's specific symptoms, lifestyle factors, and treatment goals, optimizing outcomes and improving the overall management of RA.

5. Supportive and Collaborative Care

An integrative approach to RA management fosters a collaborative and supportive care environment. It encourages open communication between healthcare providers, patients, and complementary therapy practitioners. This collaboration ensures proper coordination of treatments, addresses potential interactions or contraindications, and provides a well-rounded and comprehensive care experience. By working together, healthcare professionals can guide individuals with RA in making informed decisions about their treatment options, promoting a sense of trust, and facilitating better health outcomes.

The importance of an integrative approach to RA management cannot be overstated. By combining the strengths of conventional medicine, complementary therapies, and self-care practices, individuals with RA can experience improved symptom control, enhanced overall well-being, and a greater sense of empowerment in managing their condition.

It is essential to work closely with healthcare professionals who support and specialize in integrative medicine to develop personalized treatment plans that address the multidimensional aspects of RA. Through the integration of various treatment modalities and a collaborative approach to care, individuals with RA can optimize their treatment outcomes and achieve a higher quality of life.

Evidence-Based Research on Alternative and Complementary Therapies

Evidence-based research on alternative and complementary therapies for rheumatoid arthritis (RA) has been conducted to evaluate their effectiveness, safety, and potential benefits for individuals with the condition. While the research landscape is continually evolving, here are some key findings from existing studies:

1. Acupuncture

Several studies have suggested that acupuncture may provide pain relief and improve joint function in individuals with RA. It has been found to reduce inflammation markers, decrease pain intensity, and enhance overall well-being. However, more high-quality studies are needed to establish its long-term benefits and optimal treatment protocols.

2. Herbal Remedies

Certain herbal supplements, such as turmeric, ginger, and Boswellia serrate (frankincense), have shown promising anti-inflammatory effects in RA. They may help reduce joint pain and inflammation, although the evidence is still limited, and their safety and efficacy vary among individuals. It is crucial to consult with a healthcare professional before incorporating herbal remedies into a treatment plan.

3. Mind-Body Practices

Mindfulness-based stress reduction, meditation, and yoga have demonstrated positive effects on reducing pain, stress, and depression in individuals with RA. These practices can improve psychological well-being, enhance coping mechanisms, and promote self-management skills. They are often used as complementary therapies alongside conventional treatments.

4. Omega-3 Fatty Acids

Omega-3 fatty acids, commonly found in fish oil, have anti-inflammatory properties and may help alleviate RA symptoms. Studies have shown potential benefits in reducing joint pain and morning stiffness, improving joint function, and reducing the need for nonsteroidal anti-inflammatory drugs (NSAIDs). However, more research is needed to determine optimal dosages and long-term effects.

5. Massage Therapy

Limited research suggests that massage therapy may offer short-term pain relief and improve physical function in individuals with RA. It can help reduce muscle tension, enhance circulation, and promote relaxation. However, more rigorous studies are required to establish its efficacy and determine the best techniques and durations for RA management.

It's important to note that while these alternative and complementary therapies show promise, they should not replace conventional medical treatments for RA. They should be used as adjunct therapies under the guidance of healthcare professionals, who can provide personalized recommendations based on an individual's specific needs and medical history.

Overall, further research is needed to validate the efficacy, safety, and long-term benefits of alternative and complementary therapies for RA. It is advisable to consult with healthcare professionals and engage in shared decision-making when considering these therapies as part of an integrative treatment approach for rheumatoid arthritis.

Navigating Safety and Effectiveness: Factors to Consider

When considering complementary and alternative therapies for rheumatoid arthritis (RA), it is important to approach them with caution and consider the following factors to ensure safety and effectiveness:

1. Consult with a Healthcare Provider

Before starting any complementary or alternative therapy, consult with your healthcare provider, preferably a rheumatologist or a healthcare professional familiar with RA. They can provide guidance, assess potential interactions with your current treatments, and help you make informed decisions.

2. Research and Evidence

Look for reliable scientific research and evidence supporting the specific complementary or alternative therapy you are considering. While some therapies may have anecdotal support or historical use, it is essential to evaluate their effectiveness based on scientific studies and clinical trials.

3. Safety Considerations

Assess the safety profile of the therapy. Consider any potential side effects, interactions with medications, or contraindications based on your specific health condition. Some therapies may have risks associated with them, so it's important to understand and weigh the potential benefits against the potential harms.

4. Integration with Conventional Treatment

Complementary and alternative therapies should not replace or interfere with your prescribed medications or treatments for RA. It's crucial to ensure that the chosen therapy can be safely integrated into your overall treatment plan. Discuss this integration with your healthcare provider.

5. Professional Guidance

Seek guidance from qualified professionals or practitioners experienced in the specific therapy you are considering. They should have appropriate training and credentials in their field. Be cautious of unqualified individuals making unsubstantiated claims or offering unproven therapies.

6. Personalized Approach

Recognize that what works for one person may not work for another. Complementary and alternative therapies may have individualized effects and responses. Consider your unique health situation, preferences, and goals when assessing the suitability of a particular therapy for you.

7. Research Methodology and Quality

Evaluate the quality of the research supporting the therapy. Look for well-designed studies, randomized controlled trials, and reputable sources of information. Beware of anecdotal evidence, testimonials, or biased information that may not provide a reliable assessment of safety and effectiveness.

8. Monitoring and Evaluation

Continuously monitor your response to the therapy and any changes in your condition. Regularly communicate with your healthcare provider and discuss the therapy's effectiveness, any improvements, or potential adverse effects. This ongoing evaluation is crucial to ensure that the therapy remains safe and beneficial.

9. Cost and Accessibility

Consider the cost and accessibility of the therapy. Some complementary and alternative therapies may not be covered by insurance, and the financial burden should be evaluated alongside the potential benefits. Accessibility and availability of qualified practitioners or resources should also be taken into account.

10. Open Communication

Maintain open and honest communication with your healthcare provider about your interest in complementary and alternative therapies. Share any therapies you are considering or currently using, as well as any changes in your treatment regimen. Collaboration and transparency with your healthcare team are essential for ensuring your overall well-being.

11. Potential Interactions with Dietary Restrictions or Allergies

If the therapy involves dietary changes, supplements, or herbal remedies, consider whether they align with any dietary restrictions or allergies you may have. Ensure that the therapy does not pose any risks or conflicts with your specific dietary needs.

12. Supportive Community or Resources

Explore whether there are supportive communities or resources available for the chosen therapy. Engaging with others who have similar experiences can provide valuable insights and support throughout the journey.

Remember that complementary and alternative therapies should be seen as adjunctive approaches to conventional medical treatments for RA. They should be used in conjunction with, not as a substitute for, evidence-based medical care.

Chapter 2:

Acupuncture: Relieving Pain and Promoting Balance

Acupuncture is an ancient medical practice that originated in China and has been used for centuries to alleviate pain and promote overall well-being. It involves the insertion of thin, sterile needles into specific points on the body, known as acupuncture points. Acupuncture is based on the principle that these points are interconnected pathways through which vital energy, called Qi, flows. By stimulating these points, acupuncture aims to restore the balance and flow of Qi, facilitating the body's natural healing processes.

One of the primary applications of acupuncture is pain relief. It has been found to be particularly effective in managing various types of pain, including musculoskeletal pain, headaches, and chronic conditions such as arthritis. Acupuncture's analgesic effects are believed to be due to the release of endorphins, the body's natural pain-relieving chemicals, as well as its ability to modulate the nervous system and reduce inflammation.

In addition to pain relief, acupuncture is often used as a complementary therapy to promote overall wellness and improve various health conditions. It is believed to help regulate the body's energy flow, boost the immune system, reduce stress, and enhance mental and emotional well-being. Acupuncture is also used in conjunction with conventional medical treatments to support patients undergoing procedures like chemotherapy, where it can help alleviate treatment-related side effects.

While acupuncture has gained recognition and acceptance within the medical community, it is important to approach it with proper evaluation and in collaboration with a trained and licensed acupuncturist. The practitioner's expertise, the use of sterile needles, and adherence to safety protocols are crucial for ensuring the effectiveness and safety of acupuncture treatments.

According to the National Center for Complementary and Integrative Health (NCCIH), acupuncture can effectively help in the treatment of

- headache
- neck pain
- osteoarthritis
- low back pain and
- knee pain but warns against substituting acupuncture for traditional medical care.

Some studies also supports that acupuncture can as well assist in the treatment of:

- rheumatoid arthritis
- migraine
- tendinopathy
- nausea
- fatigue
- peripheral neuropathy

- Chemotherapy-induced and postoperative nausea and vomiting
- Dental pain
- Fibromyalgia
- Labor pain
- Menstrual cramps
- Respiratory disorders, such as allergic rhinitis
- Tennis elbow

Overall, acupuncture offers a holistic approach to pain management and well-being by addressing the body, mind, and spirit. Its ancient roots, combined with modern scientific understanding, continue to make it a popular therapy for those seeking natural and alternative methods to enhance their health and quality of life.

Demystifying Acupuncture: Principles and Practices

Acupuncture is a therapeutic practice rooted in traditional Chinese medicine (TCM) that has gained recognition and popularity worldwide. By understanding its principles and practices, we can demystify this ancient healing art.

Let's look at the followings:

A. Principles of Acupuncture:

The principles of acupuncture are rooted in traditional Chinese medicine and provide a framework for understanding its therapeutic approach.

Here are the key principles:

1. Qi (Vital Energy)

Qi is the fundamental concept in acupuncture. It is the vital energy that flows through the body along specific pathways called meridians. Qi is believed to be responsible for maintaining health and vitality. In acupuncture theory, illness is seen as a disruption or imbalance in the flow of Qi.

Here's an overview of Qi:

- **Definition:** Qi can be translated as "vital energy," "life force," or "bioenergetic force." It is considered the fundamental substance that underlies and animates all aspects of life, both within the body and in the surrounding environment.

- **Nature of Qi:** Qi is an abstract concept that represents the dynamic and interconnected aspects of existence. It is not easily measurable or quantifiable in scientific terms, but it is experienced and observed through its effects on the body, mind, and emotions.

- **Flow of Qi:** According to TCM theory, Qi flows through a network of pathways called meridians or channels. These meridians distribute Qi to all parts of the body, connecting organs, tissues, and physiological functions. Smooth and balanced Qi flow is considered essential for maintaining health, while disruptions or imbalances in Qi can lead to illness or discomfort.

- **Yin and Yang in Qi:** Qi is viewed in relation to the complementary forces of Yin and Yang. Yin represents the nourishing, cooling, and restorative aspects, while Yang represents the active, warming, and energizing aspects. A harmonious balance between Yin and Yang is necessary for the optimal functioning of Qi in the body.

- **Qi in Health and Disease:** In TCM, good health is seen as the free and balanced flow of Qi throughout the body, supporting all organ systems and maintaining overall well-being. Illness is believed to result from imbalances, blockages, or deficiencies in Qi, disrupting its flow and leading to symptoms and disease.

- **Regulation of Qi:** Acupuncture, along with other TCM practices such as herbal medicine, dietary adjustments, and qigong exercises, aims to regulate and balance Qi. By stimulating specific acupuncture points, practitioners seek to remove blockages, tonify deficiencies, and restore the smooth flow of Qi, promoting healing and restoring health.

It's important to note that the concept of Qi may not align with the Western biomedical understanding of energy. While scientific research continues to explore the physiological mechanisms underlying acupuncture and TCM, the concept of Qi remains rooted in the ancient traditions and holistic views of health and well-being.

In TCM, understanding and working with Qi is a foundational principle in diagnosing, treating, and promoting health. By addressing the flow and balance of Qi, practitioners aim to support the body's innate healing abilities and optimize overall wellness.

2. Acupuncture Points

Acupuncture points, also known as acupoints, are specific locations on the body where the flow of Qi can be accessed and influenced. These acupuncture points are believed to correspond to specific organs, tissues, or functions of the body. They are essential in acupuncture therapy as they are stimulated to restore balance and promote healing.

Here's an overview of acupuncture points:

- **Location:** Acupuncture points are located along the meridians or energy pathways in the body. These pathways connect various organs, tissues, and physiological functions. Each acupuncture point has a specific anatomical location and is identified by its unique name and number.

- **Number of Points:** There are hundreds of acupuncture points identified in traditional Chinese medicine. The exact number varies depending on the acupuncture system and tradition followed. The most commonly used acupuncture points number in the hundreds, with approximately 365 classical points and numerous additional points identified over time.

- **Point Selection:** The selection of acupuncture points is based on the individual's specific condition, symptoms, and the underlying pattern of imbalance. The acupuncturist considers the person's overall health, medical history, and diagnostic information to determine which points will be most beneficial for treatment.

- **Point Categories:** Acupuncture points are categorized based on their therapeutic effects and functions. Some points have specific indications for particular conditions or organ systems, while others have broader effects on Qi circulation, pain relief, or emotional well-being. Common categories include tonifying points, sedating points, local points, and distal points.

- **Point Stimulation:** Acupuncture points are stimulated in various ways to regulate the flow of Qi and restore balance. The primary method is needle insertion, where thin, sterile needles are gently inserted into the acupuncture points. Other techniques may include manual manipulation of the needles, heat (moxibustion), electrical stimulation (electroacupuncture), or pressure (acupressure).

- **Point Sensitivity:** Acupuncture points may vary in their sensitivity and responsiveness. Some points may be more tender or sensitive to touch, indicating an area of energy imbalance or stagnation. These points may be targeted for treatment to help restore the flow of Qi and alleviate symptoms.

- **Distal Points:** In addition to local points near the area of discomfort, acupuncturists often use distal points that are away from the affected area but have a strong therapeutic influence. These points are chosen based on their relationship to the meridians and their ability to address the underlying pattern of imbalance.

- **Individualized Treatment:** Like the selection of acupuncture points, the combination of points chosen for treatment is personalized for each individual. Acupuncturists develop a treatment plan based on the person's unique needs, adjusting the choice and combination of points as the condition and progress change over time.

Acupuncture points are considered key access points to influence the body's energy flow and restore balance. By stimulating these points, acupuncturists aim to promote healing, alleviate pain, and support overall well-being. The selection and skillful application of acupuncture points are fundamental to the practice of acupuncture therapy.

3. Meridians

Meridians are the pathways through which Qi flows in the body. They form a network connecting various organs, tissues, and physiological functions. There are twelve main meridians, each associated with specific organs or systems. These meridians have acupuncture points where Qi can be accessed and influenced.

In traditional Chinese medicine (TCM), there are twelve main meridians, also known as primary meridians or regular meridians. These meridians form a network of energy pathways through which Qi, the vital energy, flows. Each meridian is associated with specific organs and systems in the body.

Here are the twelve main meridians:

- **Lung Meridian (LU):** The Lung meridian governs the respiratory system and plays a role in immune function.
- **Large Intestine Meridian (LI):** The Large Intestine meridian is associated with the digestive system and helps eliminate waste and toxins.
- **Stomach Meridian (ST):** The Stomach meridian is related to the digestive system and is responsible for the processing and distribution of nutrients.
- **Spleen Meridian (SP):** The Spleen meridian influences digestion, metabolism, and the immune system. It is also associated with nourishing and distributing Qi.
- **Heart Meridian (HT):** The Heart meridian governs the cardiovascular system, emotional well-being, and mental clarity.

- **Small Intestine Meridian (SI):** The Small Intestine meridian is involved in the absorption and distribution of nutrients and plays a role in separating the pure from the impure.

- **Bladder Meridian (BL):** The Bladder meridian is associated with the urinary system and helps regulate fluid balance in the body.

- **Kidney Meridian (KI):** The Kidney meridian is essential for regulating water metabolism, reproductive functions, and maintaining overall vitality.

- **Pericardium Meridian (PC):** The Pericardium meridian is associated with the circulatory system and plays a role in emotional well-being and relationships.

- **Triple Burner Meridian (TB):** The Triple Burner meridian is not directly associated with a specific organ but is related to the regulation and coordination of the body's systems.

- **Gallbladder Meridian (GB):** The Gallbladder meridian is involved in the processing of fats and decision-making processes.

- **Liver Meridian (LR):** The Liver meridian influences the smooth flow of Qi and is associated with detoxification, storage of blood, and emotional balance.

These twelve main meridians form the foundation of TCM's understanding of energy flow in the body. In acupuncture, stimulating specific points along these meridians is believed to help restore balance and promote health by regulating the flow of Qi.

4. Yin and Yang

Another fundamental concept is the balance between Yin and Yang energies. They are complementary forces representing opposite and interconnected aspects of existence.

Yin represents coolness, darkness, and stillness or rest, and the feminine principle, while Yang represents warmth, light, activity and the masculine principle. Health is achieved when Yin and Yang are harmoniously in balance while illnesses arise from their disharmony.

5. Five Elements

The Five Elements theory categorizes different aspects of the body and the environment into five elemental qualities: Wood, Fire, Earth, Metal, and Water. Each element corresponds to specific organs, emotions, seasons, and other factors. The interplay and balance of these elements are essential for health and well-being.

In traditional Chinese medicine (TCM), the Five Elements theory, also known as Wu Xing, is a fundamental concept used to understand the patterns and interactions of the natural world and the human body. It provides a framework for analyzing and balancing the dynamic relationships between various phenomena.

Here's an overview of the Five Elements:

- **Wood (Mu):** Wood represents growth, expansion, and vitality. It is associated with spring, the color green, and the qualities of flexibility and creativity. In the body, Wood is related to the liver and gallbladder and influences the smooth flow of Qi and emotions.
- Fire (Huo): Fire represents warmth, transformation, and energy. It is associated with summer, the color red, and the

qualities of passion and joy. In the body, Fire is related to the heart and small intestine and governs circulation, mental clarity, and emotional well-being.

- Earth (Tu): Earth represents stability, nourishment, and grounding. It is associated with late summer or the transitional seasons, the color yellow, and the qualities of nurturing and harmony. In the body, Earth is related to the spleen and stomach, playing a role in digestion, absorption, and overall energy balance.

- Metal (Jin): Metal represents refinement, structure, and clarity. It is associated with autumn, the color white or metallic tones, and the qualities of organization and precision. In the body, Metal is related to the lungs and large intestine, governing respiration, elimination, and the immune system.

- Water (Shui): Water represents fluidity, adaptability, and wisdom. It is associated with winter, the color black or dark blue, and the qualities of depth and introspection. In the body, Water is related to the kidneys and bladder, governing water metabolism, reproductive functions, and the storage of vital essence.

The Five Elements are not seen as separate entities but as interconnected and interdependent forces. They interact with each other through a cycle of creation and control:

1. Creation Cycle: The elements follow a cycle of creation where each element generates and supports the next. Wood fuels Fire, Fire creates Earth (ash), Earth produces Metal, Metal enriches Water, and Water nourishes Wood.

2. Control Cycle: The elements also have a control cycle where each element regulates and controls the next. Wood controls

Earth by its roots, Earth absorbs Water, Water extinguishes Fire, Fire melts Metal, and Metal cuts Wood.

The Five Elements theory is applied to various aspects of TCM diagnosis, treatment, and lifestyle recommendations. It helps practitioners understand the relationships between organs, emotions, seasons, colors, and other phenomena. By identifying imbalances and disharmonies between the elements, TCM aims to restore equilibrium and promote health and well-being.

6. Holistic View

Acupuncture takes a holistic approach to health, considering the interconnectedness of the body, mind, and spirit. It recognizes that physical symptoms are often influenced by emotional, mental, and environmental factors. Acupuncture aims to restore balance and harmony in the whole person rather than just treating isolated symptoms.

7. Individualized Treatment

Acupuncture treatments are tailored to the individual's unique constitution and health condition. Practitioners take into account the person's symptoms, medical history, lifestyle, and emotional well-being to develop a personalized treatment plan. The goal is to address the underlying imbalances and support the body's self-healing mechanisms.

These principles provide a conceptual framework for understanding the principles of energy flow, balance, and interconnection within the body. They guide the diagnosis and treatment strategies employed by acupuncturists in their efforts to restore health and promote overall well-being. It is important to note that while acupuncture is widely practiced and has shown clinical benefits, the scientific understanding of its mechanisms is still evolving.

B. Practices of Acupuncture

1. Needle Insertion

During an acupuncture session, a trained practitioner inserts thin, sterile needles into specific acupuncture points on the body. The needles are typically left in place for a certain period, usually around 20 to 30 minutes.

2. Meridian Stimulation

The practitioner may manipulate the needles manually or use additional techniques like gentle twirling, heat, or electrical stimulation to enhance the therapeutic effects. The aim is to regulate the flow of Qi and restore balance in the body.

3. Individualized Treatment

Acupuncture treatments are personalized based on the individual's unique condition and needs. The practitioner conducts a thorough assessment, including a detailed consultation, examination of the tongue, pulse diagnosis, and evaluation of the overall health status.

4. Integrative Approach

Acupuncture is often used as a complementary therapy alongside conventional medicine. It can be combined with other treatment modalities, such as herbal medicine, dietary modifications, exercise, and lifestyle recommendations, to address the underlying imbalances and promote holistic healing.

5. Therapeutic Applications

Acupuncture is widely known for its effectiveness in managing pain, including musculoskeletal conditions, migraines, and menstrual cramps. It is also used to support various health conditions such as stress, anxiety, digestive disorders, fertility issues, and respiratory ailments.

6. Safety and Regulation

To ensure safety and effectiveness, it is crucial to seek treatment from a licensed and qualified acupuncturist. They adhere to strict hygiene standards, use disposable needles, and follow established guidelines and best practices.

While modern research has provided some insights into the mechanisms of acupuncture, further scientific investigation is still ongoing to fully understand its physiological effects. Acupuncture's growing popularity is attributed to its potential benefits, holistic approach, and relatively low risk of adverse effects.

Demystifying acupuncture involves appreciating its principles rooted in ancient Chinese medicine and understanding its practices as a complementary therapy that aims to restore balance, stimulate the body's innate healing capacity, and promote overall well-being.

Understanding Acupuncture's Mechanisms in Managing Rheumatoid Arthritis

Acupuncture is often used as a complementary therapy for managing rheumatoid arthritis (RA). While the precise mechanisms of how acupuncture works in RA are still being studied, several theories and observations have been proposed.

Here are some potential mechanisms by which acupuncture may help in managing RA:

- **Pain Relief**

Acupuncture is known to stimulate the release of endorphins, which are natural pain-relieving substances produced by the body. By targeting specific acupuncture points, acupuncture may help alleviate pain associated with RA by modulating the transmission of pain signals in the central nervous system.

- **Anti-Inflammatory Effects**

Studies suggest that acupuncture may have anti-inflammatory effects. It may help regulate the production and release of pro-inflammatory substances, such as cytokines and chemokines, thereby reducing inflammation in joints affected by RA.

- **Modulating the Immune Response**

Acupuncture has been found to influence the immune system by modulating immune cells and their activity. In RA, where the immune system mistakenly attacks the joints, acupuncture may help regulate immune responses and restore immune balance.

- **Enhancing Blood Circulation**

Acupuncture is believed to improve blood circulation. By enhancing blood flow to the affected joints, it may promote the delivery of nutrients, oxygen, and immune cells, while facilitating the removal of metabolic waste products and inflammatory mediators.

- **Balancing Qi Flow**

According to traditional Chinese medicine, RA is seen as an imbalance or blockage of Qi, the vital energy. Acupuncture aims to restore the smooth flow of Qi by stimulating specific acupuncture points. By doing so, it may help address the underlying energetic imbalances associated with RA.

- **Modulating Neurotransmitters**

Acupuncture may influence the release and activity of neurotransmitters, such as serotonin and norepinephrine, which play a role in pain perception, mood regulation, and immune function. By modulating these neurotransmitters, acupuncture may help alleviate pain, improve mood, and support overall well-being in individuals with RA.

It's important to note that while acupuncture has shown promising results in managing RA symptoms, it is typically used as a complementary therapy alongside conventional medical treatments. It's always recommended to consult with a qualified acupuncturist and healthcare provider to develop an integrated treatment plan that addresses individual needs and preferences.

Additionally, more research is needed to fully understand the mechanisms and effectiveness of acupuncture in managing RA.

Acupuncture Points for Targeting Arthritis Symptoms

Acupuncture offers various points that can be targeted to help manage arthritis symptoms. While the specific points used may vary depending on the individual and their specific symptoms, here are some commonly utilized acupuncture points for arthritis:

1. **Large Intestine 4 (LI4)** - Located on the web between the thumb and index finger, LI4 is a commonly used point for pain relief and reducing inflammation.

2. **Hegu (LI4 and LI11)** - LI11 is another point on the Large Intestine meridian commonly used for joint pain and inflammation. It is located at the outer end of the elbow crease. Combining LI4 and LI11 is often effective in addressing arthritis symptoms.

3. **Neiguan (PC6)** - Located on the inner forearm, about two finger-widths above the wrist crease, PC6 is known for its beneficial effects on reducing pain and inflammation. It is especially effective for wrist and hand arthritis.

4. **Zusanli (ST36)** - Situated below the kneecap, on the outer side of the leg, ST36 is a versatile point used for a wide range of conditions. It helps improve joint mobility, reduce inflammation, and enhance overall energy and vitality.

5. **Sanyinjiao (SP6)** - Located on the inner leg, about four finger-widths above the ankle bone, SP6 is commonly used for a variety of conditions, including arthritis. It helps alleviate joint pain and inflammation while promoting relaxation and balancing energy.

6. **Fengchi (GB20)** - Situated at the base of the skull, in the hollows on both sides of the neck, GB20 is often used for neck and shoulder arthritis. It helps relieve pain, stiffness, and tension in the upper body.

7. **Taichong (LV3)** - Located on the top of the foot, in the depression between the big toe and the second toe, LV3 is an important point for overall pain management. It is especially useful for addressing joint pain associated with arthritis.

It's important to note that acupuncture treatment is individualized, and the selection of specific acupuncture points will depend on the individual's unique symptoms, patterns of disharmony, and the assessment of the acupuncturist. Consulting with a qualified acupuncturist is crucial to receive personalized treatment that addresses your specific arthritis symptoms.

Acupuncture in Combination with Traditional Treatments: Optimizing Results

When it comes to managing various conditions, including arthritis, acupuncture is often used as a complementary therapy alongside traditional medical treatments. Integrating acupuncture with conventional approaches can optimize results and provide a more comprehensive approach to healthcare.

Here's how acupuncture, in combination with traditional treatments, can help optimize results:

1. **Pain Management:**
Acupuncture is well-known for its analgesic effects and can be particularly beneficial in managing pain associated with arthritis. By stimulating acupuncture points, it can help reduce pain intensity, improve pain tolerance, and enhance overall pain management. This can complement the use of pain medications or other conventional pain management techniques, allowing for better pain control and potentially reducing the reliance on medication.

2. **Reduction of Inflammation**
Acupuncture has been found to have anti-inflammatory effects, which can be advantageous in conditions characterized by inflammation such as arthritis. While disease-modifying anti-rheumatic drugs (DMARDs) and other anti-inflammatory medications are commonly prescribed, combining acupuncture with

these treatments may enhance the anti-inflammatory response and potentially reduce the dosage or side effects of medication.

3. Improved Function and Mobility

Arthritis can impact joint function and mobility, leading to stiffness, limited range of motion, and decreased quality of life. Acupuncture, in conjunction with physical therapy and rehabilitation exercises, can help improve joint mobility, reduce stiffness, and enhance overall function. The combination of therapies can provide a synergistic effect, optimizing results and promoting better physical well-being.

4. Enhanced Psychological Well-being

Dealing with chronic conditions like arthritis can have a psychological impact, leading to stress, anxiety, and depression. Acupuncture has been shown to have positive effects on mental health by promoting relaxation, reducing stress, and improving overall emotional well-being. Integrating acupuncture with psychotherapy or counseling can provide a holistic approach to address the emotional aspects of managing arthritis.

5. Individualized Treatment

Acupuncture offers a personalized approach to healthcare, taking into account the unique symptoms, patterns, and needs of each individual. By combining acupuncture with traditional treatments, a comprehensive treatment plan can be developed, tailored to the specific needs of the patient. This personalized approach can optimize results by addressing the individual's physical, emotional, and energetic imbalances.

It's important to note that integrating acupuncture with traditional treatments should be done in consultation with healthcare professionals, including both acupuncturists and medical doctors.

They can collaborate to ensure the treatments are complementary and safe, with proper coordination and monitoring of the overall healthcare plan.

By combining the strengths of acupuncture and traditional treatments, individuals with arthritis can potentially experience enhanced pain management, improved function, better overall well-being, and an optimized approach to their healthcare journey.

Integrating Acupuncture into Your Rheumatoid Arthritis Management Plan

Integrating acupuncture into your rheumatoid arthritis (RA) management plan can be a beneficial step towards optimizing your overall treatment approach.

Here are some steps to consider when integrating acupuncture into your RA management plan:

1. Consultation with Healthcare Team

Before starting acupuncture or making any changes to your treatment plan, it's crucial to consult with your healthcare team, including your rheumatologist and acupuncturist. They can provide guidance, evaluate your specific condition, and ensure that acupuncture is safe and suitable for you.

2. Find a Qualified Acupuncturist

Seek a licensed and experienced acupuncturist who has expertise in treating rheumatoid arthritis. Ask for recommendations from your healthcare team or trusted sources. Look for certifications and credentials to ensure that the acupuncturist meets professional standards.

3. Communication and Collaboration

Establish open communication between your rheumatologist and acupuncturist. Share your treatment goals, medical history, current medications, and any concerns or changes in your condition. Collaboration between both practitioners can help create an integrated and coordinated treatment plan.

4. Treatment Plan and Frequency

Work with your acupuncturist to develop a treatment plan tailored to your specific needs. Discuss the frequency of acupuncture sessions and the duration of treatment. Acupuncture treatment may initially involve more frequent sessions, followed by maintenance sessions as your condition improves.

5. Integration with Conventional Treatment

Acupuncture should complement, not replace, your conventional medical treatment for rheumatoid arthritis. Continue following your rheumatologist's recommendations, including taking prescribed medications, undergoing physical therapy, and making lifestyle modifications. Inform your healthcare team about your decision to incorporate acupuncture into your treatment plan.

6. Symptom Management

Discuss your specific RA symptoms with your acupuncturist. They can target acupuncture points known to be effective for pain relief, reducing inflammation, improving joint mobility, and addressing other symptoms associated with RA. Acupuncture sessions can be tailored to address your unique needs and priorities.

7. Long-term Monitoring and Evaluation

Regularly assess the effectiveness of acupuncture in managing your RA symptoms. Monitor changes in pain levels, joint mobility, inflammation, and overall well-being. Provide feedback to both your acupuncturist and rheumatologist to evaluate the impact of acupuncture on your treatment plan.

8. Lifestyle Modifications

In addition to acupuncture, consider incorporating other supportive measures into your daily routine. This may include maintaining a balanced diet, practicing stress management techniques, engaging in regular exercise (as recommended by your healthcare team), and getting sufficient rest.

Remember, acupuncture is a complementary therapy, and its effectiveness may vary from person to person. Results may take time, and consistency is key. Be patient and realistic in your expectations while actively participating in your overall RA management plan.

Always prioritize safety and inform your healthcare team about any changes or additions to your treatment plan. By integrating acupuncture into your RA management plan, you can potentially enhance symptom management, improve quality of life, and take a holistic approach to your well-being.

Chapter 3

The Power of Massage Therapy: Easing Joint Stiffness and Enhancing Well-being

Massage refers to the practice of manipulating and kneading the soft tissues of the body, including muscles, tendons, ligaments, and fascia. It is a hands-on technique that involves applying pressure, tension, or vibration to these tissues to promote relaxation, relieve muscle tension, improve circulation, and enhance overall well-being.

A person who has received professional training to give massages is typically referred to as a masseur (for men) or masseuse (for women) in European nations. Due to the fact that they are required to hold a license and certification, these people are frequently referred to as "licensed massage therapists" in the United States. Since they are licensed healthcare providers, they are referred to as "registered massage therapists" in several Canadian jurisdictions.

Massage can be performed by a trained massage therapist or by individuals on themselves or others. It is commonly used as a form of therapy to promote physical and mental relaxation, reduce stress, alleviate pain, and aid in the recovery from injuries or muscle imbalances. In situations where massages are performed professionally, clients can either be reclining on a massage table, sitting in a massage chair, or lying on a mat on the floor.

Massage therapy is a hands-on therapeutic technique that involves the manipulation of soft tissues in the body, including muscles, tendons, ligaments, and connective tissues. It is a holistic approach to healthcare that aims to promote relaxation, alleviate pain, reduce muscle tension, improve circulation, and enhance overall well-being.

During a massage therapy session, a trained and licensed massage therapist applies various techniques using their hands, fingers, elbows, forearms, or specialized tools to manipulate the soft tissues of the body.

These techniques can include:

- **Effleurage:** Long, sweeping strokes used to warm up the muscles and promote relaxation.
- **Petrissage:** Kneading and squeezing movements that help loosen muscle fibers, reduce tension, and improve circulation.
- **Friction:** Circular or cross-fiber movements that target specific areas to break up adhesions, reduce scar tissue, and alleviate pain.
- **Tapotement:** Rhythmic tapping or percussive movements that stimulate the muscles and invigorate the body.
- **Compression:** Steady pressure applied to specific areas to release tension and promote relaxation.

Massage therapy can be performed on a massage table or chair, with the client either fully or partially clothed depending on the techniques used and personal comfort. The therapist may use oils, lotions, or creams to reduce friction and facilitate smooth gliding of the hands over the skin.

Massage therapy is often used as a complementary therapy alongside conventional medical treatments to support various conditions such as musculoskeletal pain, stress-related disorders, sports injuries, and chronic health conditions. It is important to consult with a healthcare provider before starting massage therapy, especially if you have any underlying health conditions or concerns.

Massage therapy sessions can vary in duration, typically ranging from 30 minutes to 90 minutes or more. The therapist may use oils, lotions, or creams to reduce friction and facilitate smoother movements over the skin.

Massage is generally considered safe and can be a valuable part of a comprehensive healthcare routine. However, it is important to communicate any specific health concerns or conditions to the massage therapist before the session to ensure that appropriate techniques and pressure levels are used.

Whether received for relaxation, stress relief, pain management, or as part of a rehabilitation program, massage offers numerous benefits for both the body and mind. Its therapeutic effects can help individuals achieve a greater sense of well-being and support overall physical and mental health.

There are various types of massage, each with its own focus and benefits. Some common types of massage include:

1. Swedish Massage

This is a gentle, relaxing massage that involves long, gliding strokes, kneading, and circular motions to promote relaxation and improve circulation.

2. Deep Tissue Massage

This technique targets deeper layers of muscle and connective tissue to release chronic muscle tension and address specific areas of pain or tightness.

3. Sports Massage

Designed for athletes and active individuals, sports massage focuses on preventing and treating injuries, improving flexibility, and enhancing performance.

4. Trigger Point Therapy

This technique targets specific points of tension or "trigger points" in muscles to alleviate pain and release muscle knots or tightness.

5. Shiatsu

Originating from Japan, Shiatsu involves applying pressure to specific points along energy pathways in the body to promote balance and stimulate the body's natural healing abilities.

6. Thai Massage

This type of massage combines stretching, acupressure, and assisted yoga postures to improve flexibility, release tension, and promote relaxation.

The Therapeutic Benefits of Massage Therapy for Rheumatoid Arthritis

Massage therapy can provide several therapeutic benefits for individuals with rheumatoid arthritis (RA), a chronic autoimmune condition that causes joint inflammation and pain. While it may not cure RA, massage therapy can help manage symptoms and improve overall well-being.

Here are some specific therapeutic benefits of massage therapy for rheumatoid arthritis:

1. Pain Relief

Massage therapy can effectively alleviate pain associated with RA. The manipulation of soft tissues helps increase blood flow, relax muscles, and reduce tension around affected joints, leading to pain reduction. By stimulating the release of endorphins, the body's natural painkillers, massage therapy can provide temporary relief from RA-related pain.

2. Reduced Joint Stiffness

RA often causes joint stiffness, making movement difficult and uncomfortable. Massage therapy can help loosen and relax the muscles surrounding the affected joints, promoting increased flexibility and reducing stiffness. This can improve range of motion and make daily activities more manageable for individuals with RA.

3. Improved Circulation

Massage therapy enhances blood circulation, which is beneficial for individuals with RA. Increased circulation helps deliver oxygen and nutrients to the affected joints, supporting their health and healing. It can also aid in the removal of waste products and reduce inflammation, contributing to improved joint function.

4. Stress Reduction and Relaxation

Living with RA can be physically and emotionally stressful. Massage therapy provides a calming and nurturing environment, allowing individuals to relax, reduce stress levels, and experience a sense of well-being. This can positively impact overall mental health and help manage the emotional challenges associated with RA.

5. Enhanced Sleep Quality

Many individuals with RA struggle with sleep disturbances, such as difficulty falling asleep or staying asleep due to pain and discomfort. Massage therapy promotes relaxation and can help improve sleep quality by reducing pain, alleviating muscle tension, and inducing a state of relaxation. Better sleep can contribute to overall well-being and improved ability to cope with RA symptoms.

6. Increased Joint Mobility

Massage therapy techniques, such as gentle stretching and mobilization, can help improve joint mobility in individuals with RA. By reducing muscle tightness and promoting flexibility, massage therapy can enhance the range of motion in affected joints, making daily movements and activities easier and less painful.

7. Improved Mood and Emotional Well-being

Living with a chronic condition like RA can take a toll on mental health. Massage therapy promotes the release of endorphins, serotonin, and dopamine, which are neurotransmitters associated with feelings of well-being and happiness. This can help reduce anxiety, depression, and overall emotional distress often experienced by individuals with RA.

8. Decreased Inflammation

Massage therapy has been found to have anti-inflammatory effects. It can help reduce the production of inflammatory substances in the body and promote the release of anti-inflammatory substances, leading to a decrease in overall inflammation associated with RA.

9. Enhanced Body Awareness

Through regular massage therapy sessions, individuals with RA can develop a greater sense of body awareness. This heightened awareness can help them identify areas of tension, imbalance, or discomfort, allowing for better self-care and management of their condition.

10. Support for Overall Well-being

Massage therapy provides a holistic approach to managing RA by addressing not only physical symptoms but also the emotional and psychological aspects of living with a chronic condition. It can contribute to a sense of empowerment, self-care, and improved quality of life.

It's important to note that while massage therapy can provide relief and support for individuals with RA, it should be used as a complementary therapy alongside other RA management strategies, including medication, exercise, and lifestyle modifications. Before starting massage therapy, it is essential to consult with your healthcare team, including your rheumatologist, to ensure that it is appropriate for your specific condition and any precautions that may need to be taken.

Overall, massage therapy offers a non-invasive and drug-free approach to managing RA symptoms, providing pain relief, reducing joint stiffness, promoting relaxation, and improving overall well-being for individuals living with this chronic condition.

Different Massage Techniques for Alleviating Pain and Reducing Inflammation

There are several massage techniques that can be beneficial for alleviating pain and reducing inflammation in various conditions, including rheumatoid arthritis. Here are some massage techniques commonly used for these purposes:

1. Swedish Massage

This technique involves long, gliding strokes, kneading, and circular movements to relax muscles and improve circulation. It can help reduce muscle tension and promote overall relaxation, which can alleviate pain and inflammation.

2. Deep Tissue Massage

Deep tissue massage targets the deeper layers of muscles and connective tissues. The therapist uses slow, firm pressure and focuses on specific areas of tension or pain. This technique can help relieve chronic muscle tension, break up scar tissue, and promote blood flow to the affected area, which can reduce inflammation and relieve pain.

3. Myofascial Release

Myofascial release focuses on releasing tension in the fascia, the connective tissue that surrounds and supports muscles and other structures. The therapist applies sustained pressure and gentle stretching to release restrictions and restore normal movement. By releasing tension in the fascia, myofascial release can alleviate pain, improve mobility, and reduce inflammation.

4. Trigger Point Therapy

This technique targets specific points of muscle tension called trigger points. The therapist applies pressure to these points, which can be tender or refer pain to other areas of the body. By releasing trigger points, this technique can reduce pain, improve muscle function, and decrease inflammation in the affected area.

5. Sports Massage

Sports massage is often used to prevent and treat sports-related injuries, but it can also be beneficial for individuals with rheumatoid arthritis. It combines various techniques, including deep tissue massage and stretching, to improve circulation, relieve muscle tension, and promote flexibility. Sports massage can help reduce inflammation, alleviate pain, and enhance overall physical performance.

6. Lymphatic Drainage Massage

This gentle massage technique focuses on stimulating the lymphatic system to remove excess fluid and toxins from the body. By improving lymphatic flow, lymphatic drainage massage can help reduce swelling, inflammation, and pain associated with rheumatoid arthritis.

It's important to note that the specific massage techniques used will depend on the individual's condition, preferences, and the expertise of the massage therapist. A qualified massage therapist will assess your needs and tailor the treatment accordingly. It's recommended to consult with a licensed massage therapist who has experience working with individuals with rheumatoid arthritis to ensure that the techniques used are safe and effective for your specific situation.

Massage for Joint Mobility and Flexibility Enhancement

Massage therapy can be a valuable tool for improving joint mobility and enhancing flexibility. Here are some techniques and considerations for incorporating massage into your routine to promote joint health:

1. Swedish Massage

Swedish massage techniques involve long, gliding strokes, kneading, and circular motions to increase blood circulation and relax muscles. This type of massage can help reduce muscle tension and promote joint flexibility.

2. Range of Motion (ROM) Techniques

Massage therapists can use specific ROM techniques to target joint mobility. These techniques involve gentle stretching, bending, and rotating the joints within their normal range of motion. This helps to improve joint flexibility and increase synovial fluid circulation.

3. Deep Tissue Massage

Deep tissue massage focuses on releasing tension in the deeper layers of muscle and connective tissue. By targeting specific muscle groups around the joints, deep tissue massage can alleviate stiffness, improve joint mobility, and enhance overall flexibility.

4. Myofascial Release

Myofascial release is a technique that targets the fascia, a connective tissue surrounding muscles and joints. By applying gentle sustained pressure and stretching techniques, myofascial release can release restrictions, improve flexibility, and enhance joint mobility.

5. Active and Passive Stretching

Massage therapists can incorporate active and passive stretching into the session to further improve joint flexibility. Active stretching involves engaging the muscles surrounding the joint to promote flexibility, while passive stretching involves the therapist gently moving your limbs to stretch the muscles and increase range of motion.

6. Communication with the Therapist

It's important to communicate with your massage therapist regarding any joint issues, limitations, or discomfort you may have. They can then tailor the massage techniques to your specific needs and ensure that the pressure and movements applied are appropriate and beneficial.

7. Regular Maintenance

Consistency is key when it comes to improving joint mobility and flexibility. Incorporating regular massage sessions into your routine can provide ongoing benefits and help maintain the gains achieved. Work with your therapist to establish a suitable schedule that aligns with your goals and lifestyle.

Remember, while massage therapy can be beneficial for joint mobility and flexibility enhancement, it should not be used as a substitute for medical advice or treatment. If you have any underlying medical conditions or concerns, it's advisable to consult with a healthcare professional before pursuing massage therapy.

Choosing a Qualified Massage Therapist: Tips and Considerations

It is crucial to choose a competent massage therapist to provide a safe and successful massage experience, effective treatment, understanding of contraindications to enable him to provide suitable therapy, respect for ethics and boundaries, as this will establish trust and peace of mind.

Here are some tips and considerations to help you choose a skilled and reputable massage therapist:

1. Qualifications and Credentials

Look for a massage therapist who is licensed or certified in your area. Different regions may have specific requirements and certifications, so familiarize yourself with the standards in your location. Verify their credentials through the appropriate licensing boards or professional associations.

2. Experience and Specializations

Consider the therapist's experience and any specializations they may have. Some therapists focus on specific techniques, such as sports massage, deep tissue massage, or prenatal massage. If you have specific needs or preferences, find a therapist who has expertise in those areas.

3. Referrals and Recommendations

Seek referrals and recommendations from friends, family, or healthcare professionals. Personal experiences and word-of-mouth can provide valuable insights into the therapist's skills, professionalism, and client satisfaction.

4. Research Reviews and Testimonials

Read online reviews and testimonials to gather feedback from previous clients. This can give you an idea of the therapist's reputation and the quality of their services. However, keep in mind that individual experiences can vary, so consider multiple reviews and opinions.

5. Consultation and Communication

Schedule a consultation or speak with the therapist before your first appointment. This allows you to discuss your specific needs, concerns, and goals. A qualified therapist will listen attentively, address your questions, and tailor the massage session to meet your individual requirements.

6. Professionalism and Ethics

Ensure that the therapist maintains a high level of professionalism and adheres to ethical standards. They should prioritize your comfort, privacy, and safety throughout the session. Professionalism also includes maintaining appropriate boundaries and respecting your consent.

7. Insurance and Liability Coverage

Inquire about the therapist's insurance coverage. It is beneficial for both the therapist and the client to have liability insurance, which provides protection in the event of an injury or accident during the massage session.

8. Personal Comfort and Trust

Trust your instincts and consider your overall comfort level with the therapist. It is crucial to feel at ease, respected, and safe during the massage. If you have any reservations or discomfort, it may be better to explore other options.

Remember that finding the right massage therapist is a personal decision based on your individual needs and preferences. Take your time to research, ask questions, and evaluate your options before making a choice. A qualified and skilled massage therapist can contribute significantly to your overall well-being and massage experience.

Incorporating Massage Therapy into Your Self-Care Routine

Incorporating massage therapy into your self-care routine can provide numerous benefits for your physical and mental well-being. Here are some tips to help you integrate massage therapy into your self-care practices:

1. Set aside dedicated time

Schedule regular appointments with a massage therapist or allocate time for self-massage at home. Treat it as an essential part of your self-care routine and prioritize this time for relaxation and rejuvenation.

2. Choose the right type of massage

Explore different types of massage therapy to find what works best for you. Whether you prefer a gentle Swedish massage, a deep tissue massage for muscle tension, or a specialized technique like Thai massage or hot stone massage, select the modality that aligns with your needs and preferences.

3. Create a soothing environment

Set the mood for relaxation by creating a calm and peaceful environment. Dim the lights, play soft music, and consider using aromatherapy with essential oils to enhance the ambiance. Use comfortable pillows, blankets, or cushions to support your body during self-massage.

4. Practice mindfulness

Before starting your massage session, take a few moments to center yourself and practice mindfulness. Focus on your breath, observe any sensations in your body, and let go of any stress or tension. This can help you relax and fully engage in the massage experience.

5. Incorporate self-massage techniques

Learn simple self-massage techniques to use between professional sessions or for daily self-care. Use gentle strokes, kneading, and circular motions to target areas of tension or discomfort. Pay attention to your body's response and adjust the pressure or technique as needed.

6. Explore additional tools

Consider using massage tools such as foam rollers, massage balls, or handheld massagers to complement your self-care routine. These tools can help release muscle knots, improve circulation, and enhance the effectiveness of your self-massage practice.

7. Combine massage with other self-care activities

Integrate massage therapy with other self-care practices to create a holistic approach. For example, you can precede or follow a massage session with a warm bath, meditation, stretching exercises, or gentle yoga poses to further enhance relaxation and promote overall well-being.

8. Stay hydrated and practice self-care post-massage

Drink plenty of water before and after your massage session to support the body's natural detoxification process. After the massage, allow yourself time to rest and avoid strenuous activities to fully enjoy the benefits of the treatment.

Remember, self-care is a personal journey, and it's important to listen to your body's needs. If you have any underlying health conditions or concerns, consult with a healthcare professional before incorporating massage therapy into your self-care routine. Enjoy the rejuvenating benefits of massage therapy as you prioritize your well-being.

Chapter 4

Mind-Body Techniques: Cultivating Resilience and Managing Stress

Mind-body techniques have gained increasing recognition and popularity as powerful tools for enhancing overall well-being and managing stress. These approaches acknowledge the profound connection between the mind and the body, recognizing that the health of one directly impacts the other. By integrating the power of the mind and the wisdom of the body, mind-body techniques empower individuals to cultivate resilience, reduce stress, and achieve a greater sense of balance and harmony in their lives.

At the core of mind-body techniques is the understanding that our thoughts, emotions, and beliefs have a profound impact on our physical health and vice versa. Stress, for instance, can manifest as physical tension, compromised immune function, and various health issues. By addressing the mind and body simultaneously, mind-body techniques offer a holistic approach to wellness, providing a pathway to greater self-awareness, emotional well-being, and physical vitality.

These techniques encompass a wide range of practices that promote the integration of the mind and body, such as meditation, deep breathing exercises, yoga, tai chi, mindfulness, visualization, and more. Each technique has its unique approach, but they all share a common goal: to bring awareness to the present moment, cultivate relaxation, and foster a sense of inner balance and harmony.

Through regular practice, mind-body techniques can help individuals develop greater resilience in the face of life's challenges. They offer practical tools for managing stress, anxiety, and emotional upheavals. By cultivating mindfulness and self-awareness, individuals become better equipped to navigate the ups and downs of life with grace and ease, responding to stressors in a more constructive and empowered manner.

Furthermore, mind-body techniques have been shown to have numerous physical benefits. They can lower blood pressure, reduce heart rate, enhance immune function, improve sleep quality, alleviate pain, and promote overall physical well-being. By harmonizing the mind and body, these techniques create an optimal environment for healing and restoration.

In a world that often demands constant busyness and external focus, mind-body techniques offer a sanctuary for self-care, self-reflection, and self-empowerment. They invite individuals to slow down, tune into their inner wisdom, and reconnect with their innate capacity for healing and well-being.

Mind-body techniques encompass a wide range of practices and approaches that aim to integrate and harmonize the connection between the mind and the body. These techniques acknowledge the inherent link between our mental and emotional states and our physical well-being, recognizing that the two are intricately interconnected.

The foundation of mind-body techniques lies in the understanding that our thoughts, emotions, beliefs, and attitudes can significantly influence our physical health and vice versa. By engaging the mind and the body simultaneously, these techniques seek to promote overall well-being, enhance self-awareness, and empower individuals to take an active role in their health and healing.

Mind-body techniques encompass various disciplines and practices, including but not limited to:

- **Meditation:** Meditation involves training the mind to achieve a state of focused attention and inner stillness. It encourages mindfulness, relaxation, and the cultivation of a present-moment awareness.
- **Breathing Exercises:** Deep breathing exercises, such as diaphragmatic breathing or breath awareness, harness the power of conscious breathing to induce relaxation, reduce stress, and promote physical and mental well-being.
- **Yoga:** Yoga combines physical postures (asanas), breathing techniques (pranayama), and meditation to promote flexibility, strength, balance, and a sense of inner calm.
- **Tai Chi:** Tai Chi is a mind-body practice originating from ancient Chinese martial arts. It involves slow, gentle movements, deep breathing, and focused attention to promote relaxation, balance, and overall vitality.

Guided Imagery and Visualization: These techniques involve creating vivid mental images to evoke relaxation, healing, and positive outcomes. Guided imagery uses verbal guidance, while visualization relies on one's own imagination and intention.

- **Progressive Muscle Relaxation (PMR):** PMR involves systematically tensing and relaxing different muscle groups, promoting physical and mental relaxation, and reducing muscle tension.

- **Mindfulness-Based Stress Reduction (MBSR):** MBSR is a structured program that combines mindfulness meditation, gentle yoga, and mindfulness practices to enhance self-awareness, reduce stress, and improve overall well-being.

- **Biofeedback:** Biofeedback techniques use electronic devices to provide individuals with real-time information about their physiological processes, such as heart rate, skin temperature, or muscle tension. This feedback helps individuals learn to self-regulate these bodily functions for relaxation and stress reduction.

These are just a few examples of mind-body techniques, and the field continues to evolve with ongoing research and exploration. The common thread among these practices is the recognition that by integrating the mind and the body, individuals can cultivate self-awareness, reduce stress, enhance resilience, and promote overall well-being.

The Mind-Body Connection: Exploring the Impact of Stress on Rheumatoid Arthritis

The mind-body connection plays a significant role in the overall health and well-being of individuals, and this connection is particularly evident in the context of chronic conditions like rheumatoid arthritis (RA). Rheumatoid arthritis is an autoimmune disorder characterized by inflammation in the joints, causing pain, stiffness, and swelling. While the exact cause of RA is still not fully understood, research suggests that stress and psychological factors can influence its onset, progression, and symptom severity.

Stress, both acute and chronic, can have a profound impact on the immune system and inflammatory responses in the body. When we experience stress, the body releases stress hormones like cortisol and adrenaline, which can trigger an inflammatory response. In the case of RA, this inflammatory response can exacerbate joint inflammation and contribute to increased disease activity.

Additionally, stress can lead to unhealthy coping behaviors, such as poor sleep, sedentary lifestyle, and unhealthy dietary choices, which can further contribute to the progression of RA and worsen symptoms. Chronic stress can also disrupt the body's natural healing processes, hinder medication effectiveness, and negatively impact overall quality of life for individuals with RA.

Furthermore, the psychological impact of living with a chronic condition like RA can cause emotional distress, anxiety, and depression. These mental health factors can further contribute to increased stress levels and worsen the symptoms and outcomes of RA. Conversely, managing stress and addressing psychological well-being can positively influence the management of RA and improve overall health outcomes.

Recognizing and addressing the mind-body connection in the context of RA is essential for comprehensive treatment and management. Incorporating stress management techniques, such as relaxation exercises, meditation, deep breathing, and mindfulness, can help individuals with RA reduce stress levels, promote a sense of calm, and support overall well-being.

Additionally, seeking support from mental health professionals, joining support groups, and engaging in activities that promote emotional well-being can provide individuals with the tools and resources needed to manage stress and cope with the challenges of living with RA.

It is important to note that while stress and psychological factors can impact RA, they are not the sole causes of the condition. RA is a complex autoimmune disease with multifactorial origins. However, by addressing the mind-body connection and incorporating strategies to manage stress, individuals with RA can potentially improve their quality of life, reduce symptom severity, and enhance their overall well-being.

Meditation and Mindfulness: Calming the Mind and Easing Arthritis Symptoms

Meditation and mindfulness are powerful practices that can have a positive impact on individuals living with arthritis. Arthritis is a condition characterized by inflammation and pain in the joints, which can significantly impact a person's quality of life. While meditation and mindfulness cannot cure arthritis, they can help manage symptoms and improve overall well-being.

Meditation involves training the mind to achieve a state of focused attention and inner stillness. By practicing meditation, individuals with arthritis can learn to calm the mind and cultivate a sense of relaxation, even in the midst of physical discomfort. This can help reduce stress, which is known to exacerbate arthritis symptoms. By calming the mind and reducing stress, individuals may experience a decrease in pain perception and an improvement in their ability to cope with the challenges of arthritis.

Mindfulness is the practice of being fully present and engaged in the present moment, without judgment. By cultivating mindfulness, individuals with arthritis can develop a greater awareness of their body, thoughts, and emotions. This increased self-awareness can help them better understand their pain, recognize patterns of tension or stress, and make conscious choices about self-care and pain management.

Through mindfulness, individuals can also develop a more accepting and compassionate attitude toward their condition. Instead of fighting against pain or becoming overwhelmed by it, they can learn to approach their symptoms with kindness and self-compassion. This shift in perspective can reduce the emotional burden of arthritis and improve overall well-being.

Research has shown that regular meditation and mindfulness practice can lead to measurable improvements in pain management, physical functioning, and psychological well-being for individuals with arthritis. By incorporating these practices into their daily routine, individuals may experience reduced pain intensity, increased joint flexibility, improved sleep quality, and enhanced emotional resilience.

It is important to note that meditation and mindfulness should be seen as complementary approaches to arthritis management, alongside medical treatments and other therapies recommended by healthcare professionals. Individuals with arthritis should consult with their healthcare provider before starting any new practices, particularly if they have specific joint limitations or other health considerations.

Incorporating meditation and mindfulness into daily life can be done in various ways. It can involve setting aside dedicated time for formal meditation practice, attending mindfulness-based programs or classes, or simply integrating mindful awareness into daily activities like walking, eating, or engaging in gentle movement.

By incorporating meditation and mindfulness into their routine, individuals with arthritis can cultivate a sense of inner calm, reduce stress, and develop a greater capacity to manage their symptoms and enhance their overall well-being.

Harnessing the Power of Breathing: Deep Breathing Exercises for Relaxation

Deep breathing exercises are simple yet powerful techniques that can help induce relaxation, reduce stress, and promote a sense of calm. The way we breathe directly affects our nervous system and can influence our physical and emotional well-being. By intentionally practicing deep breathing, we can activate the body's natural relaxation response and experience its numerous benefits.

Here are a few deep breathing exercises that you can incorporate into your daily routine:

- **Diaphragmatic Breathing**

Also known as belly breathing or abdominal breathing, this technique involves breathing deeply into your diaphragm rather than shallowly into your chest. To practice diaphragmatic breathing, sit or lie down in a comfortable position. Place one hand on your abdomen, just below your ribcage, and the other hand on your chest. Take a slow, deep breath in through your nose, feeling your abdomen rise as you fill your lungs with air. Exhale slowly through your mouth, allowing your abdomen to fall. Repeat this process, focusing on the sensation of your breath filling and leaving your body.

- **4-7-8 Breathing**

This technique, popularized by Dr. Andrew Weil, combines deep breathing and breathe control. Begin by exhaling completely through your mouth. Then, close your mouth and inhale quietly through your nose to a mental count of four. Hold your breath for a count of seven. Finally, exhale completely through your mouth to a count of eight. This completes one breath. Repeat this cycle three more times. This technique can help calm the mind, reduce anxiety, and promote relaxation.

- **Box Breathing**

Box breathing is a technique that involves equal-length inhalations, holds, and exhalations, creating a square or box-like pattern. Start by inhaling slowly and deeply through your nose to a count of four. Hold your breath for a count of four. Exhale slowly and completely through your nose or mouth to a count of four. Hold your breath again for a count of four. Repeat this cycle for several minutes, focusing on the rhythm and flow of your breath.

- **Alternate Nostril Breathing**

This technique is derived from ancient yogic practices and aims to balance the flow of energy in the body. Start by sitting in a comfortable position and using your right hand. Close your right nostril with your thumb and inhale deeply through your left nostril. After completing the inhalation, release your right nostril and close your left nostril with your ring finger. Exhale slowly and completely through your right nostril. Continue the pattern by inhaling through the right nostril, closing it, and exhaling through the left nostril. Repeat this cycle for several minutes, alternating between nostrils.

These deep breathing exercises can be practiced at any time of the day, whenever you feel the need to relax, reduce stress, or center yourself. You can incorporate them into your morning routine, during breaks throughout the day, or as part of a bedtime ritual. Consistent practice can help train your body and mind to respond to stress with a calmer and more relaxed state.

Remember, deep breathing exercises are not only beneficial in the moment but can also have long-term effects on your overall well-being. By harnessing the power of your breath, you can tap into a natural tool for relaxation and promote a sense of inner peace and balance.

Guided Imagery: Enhancing Well-being and Pain Management

Guided imagery is a powerful mind-body technique that involves using your imagination to create and experience vivid mental images, sensations, and scenarios. It can be a valuable tool for enhancing overall well-being, reducing stress, and managing pain. Through guided imagery, you can harness the power of your mind to positively influence your body and emotions.

During a guided imagery session, you listen to or follow the instructions of a facilitator, a recorded audio, or a script to guide your imagination through a specific scenario or visualization. This can be done individually or in a group setting. The guided imagery may involve peaceful nature scenes, healing landscapes, or any other calming and positive imagery.

Here are some ways guided imagery can enhance well-being and pain management:

- **Relaxation**

Guided imagery induces a state of deep relaxation by engaging your senses and focusing your attention on pleasant and soothing images. This relaxation response can help reduce muscle tension, lower heart rate and blood pressure, and promote an overall sense of calm.

- **Stress Reduction**

Guided imagery provides a mental escape from daily stressors. By immersing yourself in a calming and peaceful imaginary environment, you can release stress, quiet racing thoughts, and restore a sense of inner balance.

- **Pain Management**

Guided imagery has been shown to help individuals manage and reduce pain. By redirecting your attention to positive and soothing images, you can shift your focus away from pain sensations, alter pain perception, and potentially experience a decrease in pain intensity.

- **Emotional Well-being**

Guided imagery can have a positive impact on emotional well-being by promoting relaxation, reducing anxiety, and enhancing feelings of positivity and joy. It can help you tap into your inner resources, cultivate resilience, and improve overall mood.

- **Visualization of Healing**

Guided imagery can be used to visualize and support the healing process. By envisioning your body as healthy, strong, and resilient, you can strengthen your belief in your body's ability to heal and promote a positive mindset.

- **Mind-Body Connection**

Guided imagery strengthens the connection between the mind and body, allowing you to tap into the powerful interplay between thoughts, emotions, and physical sensations. By engaging your imagination, you can create a harmonious and healing state within yourself.

To practice guided imagery, find a comfortable and quiet space where you can relax without distractions. You can use pre-recorded guided imagery audios, guided meditation apps, or scripts to guide your visualization. Close your eyes, take slow, deep breaths, and allow yourself to fully immerse in the imagery presented to you. Engage all your senses and try to experience the visualization as vividly as possible.

Guided imagery can be practiced regularly as part of a self-care routine or as needed whenever you feel the need for relaxation, stress relief, or pain management. With consistent practice, you can develop a greater ability to access a state of relaxation and tap into the healing power of your mind.

It's important to note that guided imagery complements but does not replace medical treatments or professional advice. If you have specific health concerns or conditions, consult with your healthcare provider to ensure that guided imagery is appropriate for your situation.

Incorporating guided imagery into your life can be a transformative and empowering experience. By engaging your imagination and utilizing the mind-body connection, you can enhance your well-being, manage pain, and foster a greater sense of inner peace and healing.

The Benefits of Yoga for Rheumatoid Arthritis: Poses and Modifications

Yoga is a mind-body practice that combines physical postures (asanas), breathing techniques (pranayama), and meditation. It offers numerous benefits for individuals with rheumatoid arthritis (RA) by promoting flexibility, strength, balance, and a sense of inner calm. However, it's important to approach yoga for RA with caution and make appropriate modifications to ensure a safe and comfortable practice.

Here are some of the benefits of yoga for individuals with rheumatoid arthritis and suggested modifications for specific poses:

- **Increased Flexibility**

Rheumatoid arthritis can cause stiffness and reduced flexibility in the joints. Yoga poses gently stretch the muscles and joints, helping to improve flexibility over time. However, it's crucial to avoid overstretching or forcing a pose beyond your comfortable range of motion. Modify poses as needed, using props like blocks or bolsters to support your body and prevent strain.

- **Enhanced Joint Strength**

Yoga poses that engage the muscles around the joints can help strengthen and stabilize them, reducing the risk of injury and improving overall joint function. Focus on poses that gently work the muscles without putting excessive pressure on the affected joints. For example, gentle standing poses like Warrior II or modified versions of planks can help build strength without causing strain.

- **Improved Balance**

RA can affect balance and stability, making individuals more prone to falls. Yoga poses that challenge balance, such as tree pose or modified versions of standing balances, can help improve stability over time. Utilize a wall or a chair for support if needed, gradually working towards more independent balance.

- **Stress Reduction**

Managing stress is essential for individuals with RA, as stress can exacerbate symptoms. Yoga incorporates breathing techniques and meditation, which activate the body's relaxation response and help reduce stress. Practice deep breathing exercises and incorporate moments of mindfulness and meditation into your yoga practice to enhance relaxation and stress relief.

- **Mind-Body Awareness**

Yoga encourages greater awareness of your body, including sensations, limitations, and areas of strength. This heightened self-awareness can help you listen to your body's signals and adapt your practice accordingly. Honor your limitations and modify poses as needed, avoiding any movements or positions that cause pain or discomfort.

When practicing yoga with rheumatoid arthritis, consider the following modifications and suggestions:

- Start with gentle and beginner-friendly yoga classes or videos specifically designed for individuals with arthritis or joint conditions.
- Opt for slow-paced, restorative, or gentle yoga styles, such as Hatha or Yin yoga, which focus on relaxation and gentle stretching.
- Utilize props like blankets, blocks, or bolsters to provide support and make poses more accessible and comfortable.
- Avoid putting excessive pressure on the affected joints. If a pose causes pain or discomfort, modify it or skip it altogether.
- Warm up before starting your yoga practice with gentle movements and range-of-motion exercises to prepare your body.
- Listen to your body and take breaks as needed. Resting when necessary helps prevent overexertion and reduces the risk of flare-ups.
- Work with a knowledgeable yoga instructor who has experience working with individuals with arthritis to receive personalized guidance and modifications.

Remember, it's essential to consult with your healthcare provider before starting any new exercise regimen, including yoga, to ensure it is suitable for your specific condition and overall health.

By incorporating yoga into your routine with appropriate modifications, you can experience the benefits of improved flexibility, strength, balance, stress reduction, and a greater sense of well-being while managing rheumatoid arthritis.

Chapter 5

Herbal Remedies and Supplements: Nature's Support for Joint Health

Herbal remedies and supplements refer to natural products derived from plants that are used to support health and well-being. They come in various forms, including capsules, tablets, liquids, extracts, teas, and topical preparations. These remedies and supplements contain active compounds from plants, such as herbs, flowers, roots, seeds, or leaves, which are believed to provide therapeutic benefits.

Herbal remedies have been used for centuries in traditional medicine systems, such as Ayurveda, Traditional Chinese Medicine (TCM), and Native American healing practices. They are often used to address specific health concerns, alleviate symptoms, or promote overall wellness. In recent years, there has been growing interest in using herbal remedies and supplements as complementary approaches to conventional medical treatments.

Supplements, on the other hand, typically refer to concentrated forms of specific nutrients or bioactive compounds, such as vitamins, minerals, amino acids, fatty acids, or plant extracts. They are available in the form of oral capsules, tablets, powders, or liquids and are intended to supplement the diet.

While herbal remedies and supplements are derived from natural sources, it's important to recognize that they are not regulated in the same way as pharmaceutical drugs. The quality, safety, and efficacy of herbal remedies and supplements can vary, and not all products on the market are supported by robust scientific evidence. Therefore, it's essential to choose reputable brands, consult with healthcare professionals, and be aware of potential interactions with medications or existing health conditions.

It's important to note that herbal remedies and supplements should not be used as substitutes for prescribed medications or conventional medical treatments. They should be approached with caution and used as part of a comprehensive approach to health and well-being, in collaboration with healthcare providers who can provide guidance and monitor their use.

Herbal remedies and supplements can be considered as complementary approaches for supporting joint health in individuals with rheumatoid arthritis (RA). While it's important to note that these remedies and supplements should not replace conventional medical treatments, some herbs and supplements have shown potential in reducing inflammation, relieving pain, and improving overall joint function.

Here are a few examples:

1. Turmeric

Turmeric contains a compound called curcumin, which has anti-inflammatory properties. Curcumin may help reduce joint pain and stiffness associated with RA. It can be taken as a supplement or added to food in the form of turmeric spice. However, it's important to choose a high-quality supplement with standardized curcumin content for optimal effectiveness.

2. Ginger

Ginger is another herb known for its anti-inflammatory properties. It may help alleviate joint pain and reduce inflammation in RA. Ginger can be consumed as a spice in cooking, brewed into tea, or taken in supplement form. Some individuals find relief by using ginger topically in the form of ginger oil or applying ginger poultices to affected joints.

3. Boswellia

Boswellia serrata, also known as Indian frankincense, has been traditionally used in Ayurvedic medicine for joint conditions. It contains compounds that may help reduce inflammation and improve joint mobility. Boswellia supplements are available and can be considered as an adjunct to RA management. Look for products standardized for boswellic acid content.

4. Fish Oil

Fish oil supplements, rich in omega-3 fatty acids (such as EPA and DHA), have shown promise in reducing inflammation and improving symptoms in RA. Omega-3 fatty acids can help decrease joint pain and stiffness. It's important to choose high-quality fish oil supplements derived from sources such as wild-caught fatty fish.

5. Devil's Claw

Devil's claw is an herb with anti-inflammatory properties that may provide pain relief in RA. It has been used traditionally to manage joint pain and improve mobility. Devil's claw supplements are available in capsule or tablet form.

6. Echinacea (*Echinacea purpurea*)

Echinacea is an herb commonly used to support immune function. It is believed to have immunomodulatory and anti-inflammatory properties. While it is primarily used for conditions like colds and respiratory infections, some studies suggest that echinacea may also have potential benefits for autoimmune conditions like rheumatoid arthritis. Echinacea supplements are available in different forms, such as capsules, tablets, and liquid extracts.

It's crucial to consult with your healthcare provider or rheumatologist before incorporating any herbal remedies or supplements into your RA management plan. They can provide personalized guidance, evaluate potential interactions with your current medications, and monitor your overall health.

Remember, herbal remedies and supplements should not be viewed as standalone treatments for RA. They can be considered as part of a comprehensive approach that includes conventional medical treatments, exercise, a balanced diet, and lifestyle modifications. Working collaboratively with your healthcare team will ensure a safe and effective approach to managing your RA symptoms.

Exploring the Anti-Inflammatory Properties of Herbal Remedies

Herbal remedies have been recognized for their potential anti-inflammatory properties, and many herbs have been studied for their effects on reducing inflammation in the body. Chronic inflammation is associated with various health conditions, including rheumatoid arthritis, cardiovascular disease, and certain types of cancer. Here are some herbal remedies that are known for their anti-inflammatory properties:

1. **Turmeric (*Curcuma longa*)**

Curcumin, the active compound in turmeric, has been extensively studied for its potent anti-inflammatory effects. It inhibits various inflammatory pathways in the body, including the NF-kB pathway, which is involved in the regulation of inflammatory responses. Curcumin has shown promise in reducing inflammation in conditions such as rheumatoid arthritis, inflammatory bowel disease, and osteoarthritis.

2. **Ginger (*Zingiber officinale*)**

Ginger contains gingerols and shogaols, which possess anti-inflammatory properties. Ginger has been studied for its ability to inhibit pro-inflammatory mediators and reduce inflammation in conditions like osteoarthritis, rheumatoid arthritis, and gastrointestinal disorders.

3. **Boswellia (*Boswellia serrata*)**

Boswellic acids found in Boswellia have demonstrated anti-inflammatory effects by inhibiting certain enzymes involved in inflammation, such as 5-lipoxygenase and leukotrienes. Boswellia has been traditionally used for its anti-inflammatory properties and has shown promise in reducing inflammation and relieving symptoms in conditions like osteoarthritis and rheumatoid arthritis.

4. **Green Tea (*Camellia sinensis*)**

Green tea contains catechins, particularly epigallocatechin gallate (EGCG), which have potent anti-inflammatory properties. Green tea has been shown to inhibit inflammatory pathways and reduce inflammation in various studies. It may have beneficial effects on conditions such as cardiovascular disease, inflammatory bowel disease, and certain types of cancer.

5. Garlic (*Allium sativum*)

Garlic contains sulfur compounds, including allicin, that possess anti-inflammatory properties. Garlic has been found to inhibit the production of pro-inflammatory substances and modulate immune responses. It may have protective effects against chronic inflammation-related conditions, such as cardiovascular disease and certain cancers.

6. Echinacea (*Echinacea purpurea*)

Echinacea is a herb commonly used to support immune function and has been traditionally used to treat colds and respiratory infections. It contains various bioactive compounds, including polysaccharides and alkamides, which have immune-stimulating and anti-inflammatory properties.

Echinacea has shown promise in modulating immune responses and reducing inflammation. While its exact mechanisms of action are not fully understood, some studies suggest that Echinacea may inhibit pro-inflammatory cytokines and promote anti-inflammatory effects. It has been studied in conditions such as upper respiratory infections, bronchitis, and inflammatory skin conditions.

7. Devil's Claw (*Harpagophytum procumbens*)

Devil's Claw is an herb native to southern Africa and has a long history of traditional use for its anti-inflammatory properties. It contains harpagosides, which are believed to be responsible for its medicinal effects. Devil's Claw has been studied for its potential in reducing inflammation and relieving pain, particularly in conditions such as osteoarthritis and lower back pain. It may work by inhibiting the production of pro-inflammatory mediators, such as cytokines and prostaglandins.

It's important to note that while these herbal remedies have demonstrated anti-inflammatory properties in studies, they may not be a substitute for medical treatments. It's always recommended to consult with a healthcare professional before incorporating herbal remedies into your health regimen, especially if you have specific health conditions or are taking medications.

Additionally, the quality and standardization of herbal supplements can vary, so it's important to choose reputable brands and follow recommended dosages. Integrating these herbal remedies into a healthy lifestyle, including a balanced diet, regular exercise, stress management, and adequate sleep, can contribute to an overall anti-inflammatory approach to health.

Dietary Supplements for Rheumatoid Arthritis: Omega-3 Fatty Acids, Glucosamine, and Chondroitin

Dietary supplements can be used as complementary approaches for managing symptoms of rheumatoid arthritis (RA). While they should not replace prescribed medications or medical advice, some supplements have shown potential benefits in reducing inflammation, improving joint health, and relieving symptoms.

Here are a few commonly used dietary supplements for rheumatoid arthritis:

1. Omega-3 Fatty Acids

Omega-3 fatty acids, particularly eicosapentaenoic acid (EPA) and docosahexaenoic acid (DHA), have anti-inflammatory properties. They can help reduce joint inflammation and alleviate symptoms such as pain and stiffness. Omega-3 fatty acids are commonly found in fatty fish like salmon, mackerel, and sardines. For those who don't consume enough fish, omega-3 supplements derived from fish oil or algae are available.

2. Glucosamine

Glucosamine is a natural compound found in the body, particularly in joint cartilage. It is commonly used as a supplement to support joint health and reduce pain in conditions like osteoarthritis and rheumatoid arthritis. Glucosamine supplements are often derived from shellfish shells and are available in various forms, including glucosamine sulfate, glucosamine hydrochloride, and N-acetyl-glucosamine. While evidence for its effectiveness in RA is limited, some individuals report symptom improvement with glucosamine supplementation.

3. Chondroitin

Chondroitin is another compound found in joint cartilage. It is often combined with glucosamine in dietary supplements to support joint health and reduce pain. Chondroitin may help protect cartilage and inhibit enzymes that contribute to joint damage. While the evidence on chondroitin's effectiveness in RA is mixed, it may provide symptomatic relief for some individuals.

It's important to note that the effectiveness of these supplements can vary from person to person, and results may take time to be noticeable. It's recommended to consult with a healthcare professional before starting any new dietary supplement, as they can provide personalized guidance, consider potential interactions with medications, and monitor your overall health.

Furthermore, it's important to choose reputable brands when purchasing supplements, as quality can vary. Be aware that supplements are not regulated in the same way as medications, so it's important to do thorough research and choose products that have undergone third-party testing for purity and quality.

Incorporating these dietary supplements should be part of a comprehensive approach to managing RA, which may include prescribed medications, regular exercise, a balanced diet, stress management, and regular check-ups with your healthcare provider.

Navigating the World of Supplements: Safety, Quality, and Potential Interactions

When considering dietary supplements, it's important to navigate the world of supplements with caution and be mindful of safety, quality, and potential interactions.

Safety should be a top priority when it comes to using dietary supplements. While they are generally regarded as safe, improper use or excessive doses can carry risks. Supplements may interact with medications or exacerbate certain health conditions. Consulting with a healthcare professional before starting any new supplement is crucial, especially if you have underlying health conditions, take medications, are pregnant or breastfeeding, or have scheduled surgery.

Quality is another crucial aspect to consider. The supplement industry is not as strictly regulated as the pharmaceutical industry, leading to variability in quality and purity among different brands and products. It's important to choose reputable brands that follow good manufacturing practices (GMP) and undergo third-party testing for quality assurance. Look for certifications or labels such as the United States Pharmacopeia (USP) seal or NSF International certification.

When making supplement choices, it's important to rely on scientific evidence and research. While testimonials and anecdotal reports can be informative, they should not be the sole basis for decision-making. Look for supplements that have been studied in well-designed clinical trials, and pay attention to the strength of evidence supporting their effectiveness.

Potential interactions with medications are a crucial consideration. Supplements can interact with medications, potentially reducing their effectiveness or causing adverse effects. Inform your healthcare provider about all the supplements you are taking or planning to take, including herbal remedies and over-the-counter supplements. They can help assess potential interactions and provide guidance on appropriate dosages and timing.

Reliable information sources are essential for making informed decisions about supplements. Be cautious of misleading or inaccurate information. Rely on reputable sources such as government health agencies, professional healthcare organizations, and well-established research institutions. These sources provide evidence-based information and can help you make informed decisions about supplements.

It's important to remember that everyone's body and health needs are unique. What works for one person may not work the same way for another. It's important to listen to your body, pay attention to any changes or side effects, and consult with a healthcare professional who can provide personalized guidance based on your specific circumstances.

Dietary supplements should not be seen as substitutes for a healthy diet or prescribed medications. They should be viewed as complementary approaches that can support overall health and well-being. Incorporate supplements as part of a comprehensive approach that includes a balanced diet, regular exercise, adequate rest, stress management, and appropriate medical care.

Working with a Healthcare Professional: Developing a Personalized Supplement Plan

Working with a healthcare professional is crucial when developing a personalized supplement plan. Here are some key points to consider when collaborating with a healthcare professional:

1. Consultation

Schedule an appointment with a qualified healthcare professional, such as a doctor, registered dietitian, or naturopathic doctor, who is knowledgeable about supplements and their potential interactions. During the consultation, provide a comprehensive medical history, including any current health conditions, medications, allergies, and previous supplement use.

2. Individual Assessment

The healthcare professional will conduct an individual assessment to understand your specific needs and goals. They may ask questions about your diet, lifestyle, exercise routine, and symptoms related to your health condition. This assessment will help them tailor a supplement plan that aligns with your unique circumstances.

3. Evidence-Based Recommendations

A knowledgeable healthcare professional will base their recommendations on scientific evidence and research. They will consider the available evidence for different supplements, their potential benefits, and any potential risks or interactions. They can guide you on the appropriate dosage, timing, and duration of supplementation.

4. Integration with Current Treatment

If you are already undergoing treatment for a health condition, the healthcare professional will consider how supplements can complement or interact with your current treatment plan. They will ensure that the supplements do not interfere with the efficacy of prescribed medications and address any concerns you may have.

5. Monitoring and Follow-Up

Regular monitoring and follow-up with the healthcare professional are essential. They can assess your progress, make adjustments to the supplement plan if necessary, and address any new concerns or questions that arise. They may also recommend regular blood tests or other assessments to monitor your health status.

6. Open Communication

Maintain open and honest communication with your healthcare professional. Inform them of any changes in your health, including new symptoms or the addition of other medications or supplements. This information will help them provide the most accurate guidance and ensure your safety.

Remember that a personalized supplement plan is part of a comprehensive approach to health and should be integrated with other lifestyle factors such as a balanced diet, regular exercise, stress management, and adequate rest. The supplement plan should be periodically reassessed and adjusted based on your evolving health needs.

By collaborating with a healthcare professional, you can develop a personalized supplement plan that is safe, effective, and tailored to your specific circumstances, ultimately supporting your overall health and well-being.

Chapter 6

Heat and Cold Therapy: Soothing Pain and Reducing Inflammation

Heat therapy, also known as thermotherapy, refers to the therapeutic use of heat to provide pain relief, promote healing, and relax muscles. It involves applying heat to specific areas of the body, either locally or in the form of whole-body treatments. Heat therapy can be administered through various methods such as warm compresses, heating pads, warm baths, or heated gel packs.

Cold therapy, also known as cryotherapy, involves the therapeutic use of cold to alleviate pain, reduce inflammation, and numb the affected area. Cold therapy can be applied locally to specific body parts or used as a whole-body treatment. Common methods of cold therapy include ice packs, cold compresses, cold baths or showers, and ice massage.

Both heat and cold therapy work by affecting the body's blood vessels and nerve endings. Heat causes blood vessels to dilate, increasing blood flow and delivering nutrients and oxygen to the area. It also helps relax muscles and provides a soothing sensation. Cold, on the other hand, causes blood vessels to constrict, reducing blood flow and decreasing inflammation and swelling. Cold therapy numbs the nerve endings, providing pain relief and reducing sensations of discomfort.

The choice between heat and cold therapy depends on the type of injury or condition being treated. Heat therapy is generally more suitable for chronic conditions, muscle aches, and stiffness, while cold therapy is typically used for acute injuries, swelling, and acute pain relief.

It's important to note that heat and cold therapy should be used with caution and following appropriate guidelines to avoid potential burns, frostbite, or other adverse effects. Consulting a healthcare professional is recommended, especially if you have underlying health conditions or are unsure about the suitability of these therapies for your specific situation.

Understanding when to use heat or cold therapy and how they work can help optimize their effectiveness in soothing pain and promoting healing.

Heat Therapy

1. **Vasodilation and Increased Blood Flow:** Applying heat to an area causes blood vessels to dilate, leading to increased blood circulation. This helps deliver oxygen, nutrients, and immune cells to the affected area, promoting healing and tissue repair.
2. **Muscle Relaxation:** Heat therapy can help relax muscles and reduce muscle spasms. It can also improve flexibility and range of motion.
3. **Pain Relief:** Heat can provide temporary pain relief by blocking pain signals and reducing the transmission of pain to the brain.

Heat therapy is typically beneficial for:

- Muscular aches and stiffness
- Arthritis pain
- Muscle spasms
- Chronic pain conditions
- Before engaging in activities that may cause muscle strain

Common methods of heat therapy include:

- Warm compresses or heating pads
- Warm baths or showers
- Warm gel packs or wraps
- Hot water bottles

It is important to use caution when applying heat therapy to avoid burns or excessive heat exposure. Always follow the instructions provided with heating devices and check the skin periodically during the treatment.

Cold Therapy

1. **Vasoconstriction and Reduced Blood Flow:** Applying cold to an area causes blood vessels to constrict, reducing blood flow to the area. This can help decrease inflammation and swelling.
2. **Numbing Sensation:** Cold therapy numbs the nerve endings in the affected area, reducing pain and providing immediate relief.
3. **Reduced Metabolic Activity:** Cold therapy can slow down metabolic processes, reducing cellular damage and minimizing the release of inflammatory substances.

Cold therapy is typically beneficial for:

- Acute injuries, such as sprains, strains, or bruises
- Swelling and inflammation
- Headaches or migraines
- Dental pain or swelling

Common methods of cold therapy include:

- Ice packs or cold gel packs
- Cold compresses or cold towels
- Cold baths or showers
- Ice massage

To avoid cold-induced injuries, it is essential to wrap the cold pack or ice in a thin cloth or towel before applying it to the skin. This helps prevent direct contact and provides a barrier against extreme cold.

It is worth noting that heat and cold therapy are generally considered safe for short-term use. However, if you have a pre-existing medical condition or are uncertain about the suitability of these treatments for your specific situation, it is recommended to consult a healthcare professional for guidance.

In summary, heat and cold therapy are effective methods for soothing pain and reducing inflammation. Heat therapy promotes increased blood flow, muscle relaxation, and pain relief, while cold therapy induces vasoconstriction, numbs the affected area, and reduces swelling. Understanding the appropriate use of these therapies and employing them correctly can contribute to a more comfortable and effective pain management approach.

Harnessing the Therapeutic Effects of Heat: Hot Packs, Warm Showers, and Paraffin Wax Baths

Harnessing the therapeutic effects of heat through hot packs, warm showers, and paraffin wax baths can provide soothing and therapeutic benefits for various conditions. These methods are commonly used in heat therapy, also known as thermotherapy, to promote relaxation, relieve pain, and improve circulation. Let's explore each of these techniques in more detail:

1. Hot Packs

Hot packs are portable devices or pads that can be heated and applied to specific areas of the body. They are filled with materials such as gel or grains that retain heat. Hot packs can provide localized warmth and are commonly used to alleviate muscle tension, stiffness, and mild to moderate pain.

The heat from hot packs promotes vasodilation, increasing blood flow to the area and helping to relax muscles. They can be easily applied to various body parts, such as the neck, back, shoulders, or joints. It's important to follow the instructions provided with the hot packs to avoid overheating and potential burns.

2. Warm Showers

Warm showers are a convenient and accessible way to harness the therapeutic effects of heat. A warm shower can help relax muscles, relieve stress, and provide general relaxation benefits. The warm water promotes blood circulation and may help alleviate muscle tension, joint stiffness, and mild pain.

Additionally, warm showers can have a calming effect on the mind and help promote a sense of well-being. They can be particularly beneficial after physical activity or as part of a bedtime routine to enhance relaxation and improve sleep quality.

3. Paraffin Wax Baths

Paraffin wax baths involve immersing a body part, typically hands or feet, into a bath of melted paraffin wax. The wax is heated to a comfortable temperature and creates a warm and soothing environment. The body part is dipped multiple times into the wax, creating layers that provide insulation and retain heat.

Paraffin wax baths are commonly used in the treatment of arthritis, joint pain, and conditions affecting the hands or feet. The heat from the wax helps improve blood circulation, relax muscles, reduce joint stiffness, and promote pain relief. The wax also has a moisturizing effect on the skin, leaving it soft and supple.

It's important to ensure that the wax is at a safe temperature before immersing the body part and to follow the recommended guidelines for duration and frequency of use.

When using heat therapy techniques such as hot packs, warm showers, or paraffin wax baths, it's essential to consider individual comfort levels and any specific recommendations or precautions provided by healthcare professionals. These methods can provide effective and convenient ways to harness the therapeutic benefits of heat for relaxation, pain relief, and improved well-being.

The Power of Cold Therapy: Ice Packs and Cold Compresses for Pain Relief

Cold therapy, also known as cryotherapy, is a powerful technique for pain relief and reducing inflammation. Ice packs and cold compresses are commonly used in cold therapy to provide localized cooling and therapeutic benefits.

Let's explore how these methods work and their applications:

- **Ice Packs**

Ice packs are portable devices filled with ice or a gel that can be frozen and applied to specific areas of the body. They provide direct cooling to the affected area and are widely used to reduce pain and inflammation caused by acute injuries, such as sprains, strains, bruises, or swelling.

When applied to the skin, ice packs cause vasoconstriction, narrowing blood vessels in the area. This helps reduce blood flow, inflammation, and swelling, which can alleviate pain and promote healing. Ice packs are particularly effective in the immediate aftermath of an injury to help minimize swelling and manage pain.

It's important to wrap the ice pack in a thin cloth or towel before applying it to the skin to prevent direct contact and protect the skin from ice burn. Ice therapy is typically recommended for short durations, typically around 15-20 minutes at a time, with breaks in between.

- **Cold Compresses**

Cold compresses are similar to ice packs but can be created using simple materials like a clean cloth or towel soaked in cold water or chilled in the refrigerator. They can also be used as an alternative to ice packs for providing cooling relief.

Cold compresses work in a similar way to ice packs by reducing blood flow, inflammation, and pain. They are commonly used for a variety of conditions, including headaches, dental pain, insect bites, and minor skin irritations. They are also useful in managing chronic conditions with intermittent flare-ups or for general pain relief.

Cold compresses can be applied directly to the affected area and held in place for 10-15 minutes. Repeating the application as needed can help maintain the desired cooling effect.

It's worth noting that cold therapy should not be applied directly to open wounds or areas with compromised circulation. Individuals with conditions such as Raynaud's disease or hypersensitivity to cold should exercise caution and consult a healthcare professional before using cold therapy.

Cold therapy with ice packs and cold compresses can be an effective and easily accessible method for pain relief, reducing inflammation, and managing acute injuries. When used correctly and with appropriate precautions, these techniques can provide comfort and support the body's natural healing process.

Balancing Heat and Cold: Finding the Optimal Approach for Your Symptoms

Finding the optimal approach for managing symptoms with heat and cold therapy requires understanding your specific symptoms, the nature of your condition or injury, and consulting with a healthcare professional if needed. While heat therapy and cold therapy offer distinct benefits, there are situations where a combination of both or alternating between them may be beneficial.

Here are some general guidelines to consider:

1. Acute Injuries

In the immediate aftermath of an acute injury, such as a sprain, strain, or bruise, cold therapy is often recommended to reduce swelling, inflammation, and pain. Applying an ice pack or cold compress for 15-20 minutes at a time, with intervals for the skin to warm up, can help manage acute symptoms. After the initial swelling subsides, heat therapy can be introduced to promote blood flow and relaxation.

2. Chronic Conditions and Inflammation

For chronic conditions characterized by ongoing inflammation, such as arthritis or tendonitis, heat therapy can be beneficial. Heat can help relax muscles, improve circulation, and reduce stiffness. Warm showers, heating pads, or warm compresses can provide relief. However, if there is an acute flare-up within a chronic condition, applying cold therapy initially may help manage the acute symptoms.

3. Muscle Tension and Spasms

Heat therapy is generally effective for relaxing muscles, relieving tension, and reducing muscle spasms. Applying heat through warm showers, hot packs, or paraffin wax baths can help relax tight muscles and promote flexibility. However, if there is acute inflammation accompanying muscle spasms, using cold therapy first may help reduce swelling before transitioning to heat therapy.

4. Personal Preference and Comfort

It's important to consider personal comfort and preference when choosing between heat and cold therapy. Some individuals may find one therapy more soothing or effective for their specific symptoms. Experimenting with both heat and cold therapy can help determine what works best for you.

Remember, these guidelines are general in nature, and individual responses to heat and cold therapy may vary. It's always advisable to consult with a healthcare professional, such as a doctor, physical therapist, or sports medicine specialist, to get personalized recommendations based on your specific condition or injury. They can provide guidance on the optimal approach and help tailor a treatment plan that suits your needs.

Additionally, it's important to listen to your body and adjust the duration and frequency of heat or cold therapy based on your comfort levels. If you experience persistent or worsening symptoms, it's recommended to seek medical advice for further evaluation and management.

Combining Heat and Cold Therapy with Other Rheumatoid Arthritis Treatments

Combining heat and cold therapy with other rheumatoid arthritis (RA) treatments can provide a comprehensive approach to managing symptoms and promoting overall well-being. RA is a chronic autoimmune condition that causes joint inflammation and can lead to pain, stiffness, and reduced mobility. While heat and cold therapy can offer symptomatic relief, it's important to note that they are typically used as adjunct therapies and should be integrated into a broader treatment plan prescribed by a healthcare professional.

Here are some considerations for combining heat and cold therapy with other RA treatments:

1. Medications

Heat and cold therapy can be used in conjunction with medications prescribed for RA management, such as nonsteroidal anti-inflammatory drugs (NSAIDs), disease-modifying antirheumatic drugs (DMARDs), or biologic agents. These medications help reduce inflammation, pain, and slow the progression of the disease. Heat and cold therapy can be employed as complementary approaches to help alleviate localized symptoms and improve comfort.

2. Physical Therapy

Physical therapy plays a crucial role in managing RA by improving joint function, flexibility, and strength. Heat and cold therapy can be integrated into physical therapy sessions to enhance their effectiveness. For example, heat therapy can be applied before exercise or stretching to warm up muscles and joints, while cold therapy can be used after therapy to reduce post-exercise inflammation and manage pain.

3. Splints and Supports

Heat therapy can be utilized in conjunction with splints, braces, or supports prescribed by healthcare professionals to manage joint pain and stiffness. Applying heat before wearing these devices can help relax muscles and promote joint mobility. Cold therapy can be applied after wearing the devices to reduce any inflammation or swelling that may occur.

4. Lifestyle Modifications

In addition to medical treatments, lifestyle modifications can significantly impact RA management. Heat and cold therapy can be employed as part of self-care practices. For example, taking warm showers or using heating pads in the morning can help alleviate morning stiffness. Cold therapy can be used as needed to manage acute flare-ups or reduce joint swelling.

5. Stress Management

Stress can exacerbate RA symptoms. Incorporating relaxation techniques, such as warm baths or warm compresses, can provide a calming effect and aid in stress management. Similarly, cold therapy can be used to relieve tension headaches or promote relaxation during times of stress.

It's crucial to discuss the integration of heat and cold therapy with other treatments with your healthcare provider or rheumatologist. They can provide personalized guidance, ensure that heat and cold therapy align with your overall treatment plan, and help monitor your condition's progress. Additionally, they can assist in determining the appropriate duration, frequency, and application techniques to maximize the benefits of heat and cold therapy while considering any potential contraindications or precautions specific to your condition.

Practical Tips for Incorporating Heat and Cold Therapy into Your Daily Routine

Incorporating heat and cold therapy into your daily routine can provide ongoing relief and help manage symptoms effectively. Here are some practical tips to help you incorporate these therapies into your daily life:

1. Establish a Routine

Set aside specific times during the day to incorporate heat or cold therapy into your routine. For example, you might choose to apply heat therapy in the morning to ease morning stiffness or cold therapy after physical activity to manage inflammation. Consistency is key in experiencing the benefits of these therapies.

2. Use Convenient Methods

Choose heat and cold therapy methods that are convenient and easily accessible for you. This could include using heating pads or gel packs that can be warmed in the microwave, or keeping ice packs or cold compresses in the freezer for quick access.

3. Preemptive Use

In some cases, using heat therapy before engaging in activities that may aggravate your symptoms can be beneficial. For instance, if you experience joint pain while exercising, applying heat to the affected area beforehand may help warm up the muscles and improve flexibility.

4. Post-Activity Recovery

After physical activity or strenuous exercise, cold therapy can be helpful to manage post-workout inflammation and prevent excessive swelling. Applying an ice pack or cold compress to the affected area for 15-20 minutes can aid in reducing any potential inflammation.

5. Combine with Relaxation Techniques

Incorporate heat or cold therapy into relaxation techniques to enhance their effects. For example, while practicing deep breathing exercises or meditation, you can use a warm compress on your neck or a cold compress on your forehead to promote relaxation and stress relief.

6. Adapt to Your Lifestyle

Choose heat and cold therapy methods that fit well with your lifestyle. If you prefer warm baths, allocate time for a soothing soak in the evening. If you spend long hours at a desk, consider using a heated pad on your lower back or a cold pack on your wrists during breaks.

7. Safety First

Ensure that you follow safety guidelines when using heat and cold therapy. Protect your skin from direct contact with hot or cold sources by using a thin cloth or towel as a barrier. Monitor your skin's response during treatment and discontinue if you experience any adverse reactions.

8. Seek Professional Guidance

If you're unsure about the most effective ways to incorporate heat and cold therapy into your routine, consult with a healthcare professional, such as a physical therapist or rheumatologist. They can provide personalized recommendations based on your specific condition and needs.

Remember that while heat and cold therapy can offer relief, they are typically used as part of a comprehensive treatment plan for managing specific conditions. It's important to follow the guidance of your healthcare provider and incorporate heat and cold therapy in a manner that aligns with your overall treatment goals.

Chapter 7
Hydrotherapy: Immersion for Joint Relief and Increased Mobility

Hydrotherapy is a therapeutic approach that utilizes water for the treatment of various health conditions and the promotion of overall well-being. It encompasses a wide range of techniques and practices, including the use of water in different forms, temperatures, and pressures to achieve specific therapeutic effects.

Hydrotherapy can be practiced in different settings, such as specialized hydrotherapy clinics, spa facilities, or even at home. It is often conducted under the guidance of healthcare professionals, such as physical therapists or hydrotherapists, who tailor the treatment to the individual's needs and condition.

Here are some common forms of hydrotherapy:

1. Immersion Baths

Immersion baths involve soaking in water, either partially or fully, to obtain therapeutic benefits. These baths can be performed in various temperatures, ranging from warm to cold, depending on the desired effect. Examples include warm baths for relaxation and pain relief or cold baths for stimulating circulation and reducing inflammation.

2. Contrast Hydrotherapy

Contrast hydrotherapy involves alternating between hot and cold water treatments to promote circulation and enhance healing. This technique typically involves immersing the body or specific body parts alternately in hot and cold water or applying hot and cold compresses to the affected areas.

3. Whirlpool Baths

Whirlpool baths combine water immersion with the addition of water jets or bubbles to provide massaging and therapeutic effects. The water movement and pressure from the jets help promote relaxation, improve blood circulation, and reduce muscle tension.

4. Underwater Massage

Underwater massage involves the application of massage techniques while the individual is immersed in water. The buoyancy of water combined with the therapeutic manipulation of the massage therapist can help relax muscles, relieve tension, and improve joint mobility.

5. Aquatic Exercises

Aquatic exercises refer to various forms of physical exercises performed in water. The buoyancy of water reduces the impact on the joints, making it an ideal environment for individuals with joint conditions or those seeking low-impact exercise. Water resistance can also provide gentle resistance training to strengthen muscles and improve overall fitness.

Hydrotherapy can benefit various conditions, including musculoskeletal disorders, chronic pain, arthritis, sports injuries, and certain neurological conditions. It can help reduce pain, promote relaxation, improve circulation, increase joint mobility, and facilitate overall physical and mental well-being.

It's important to note that while hydrotherapy can be beneficial, it may not be suitable for everyone. It's recommended to consult with a healthcare professional before starting hydrotherapy to determine if it's appropriate for your specific condition and to receive proper guidance on techniques, duration, and frequency of treatments.

Hydrotherapy, also known as water therapy, involves the therapeutic use of water to promote joint relief, increased mobility, and overall well-being. Immersion in water provides a unique environment that offers buoyancy, resistance, and temperature control, making it an effective modality for various conditions.

Here's how hydrotherapy can benefit joint health and mobility:

1. Buoyancy

Immersion in water reduces the effects of gravity on the body, creating a buoyant environment that relieves pressure on the joints. This buoyancy helps support the body's weight, making movement easier and reducing the impact on the joints. It allows for gentle exercises and movements that may be challenging or painful on land.

2. Reduced Joint Stress

Water provides a low-impact environment, making it ideal for individuals with joint conditions such as arthritis or those recovering from injuries. The water's buoyancy and support help reduce stress on the joints, allowing for pain-free movement and exercise. This can help improve joint flexibility, reduce stiffness, and promote joint mobility.

3. Resistance Training

The resistance provided by water during hydrotherapy exercises can help strengthen muscles around the joints. Water resistance is proportional to the speed and surface area of movement, making it an adjustable and customizable form of resistance training. Strengthening the muscles can provide stability and support to the joints, improving overall joint function.

4. Warm Water Therapy

Warm water used in hydrotherapy can have a relaxing and soothing effect on the body. The warmth helps promote muscle relaxation, increases blood circulation, and can provide pain relief. It can help reduce joint stiffness, relieve muscle tension, and enhance flexibility. Warm water therapy can be particularly beneficial for individuals with conditions such as rheumatoid arthritis or fibromyalgia.

5. Aerobic Conditioning

Hydrotherapy can also be used for aerobic conditioning, allowing individuals to engage in cardiovascular exercises in a low-impact environment. Water aerobics or swimming can improve cardiovascular fitness, strengthen muscles, and promote overall physical well-being without putting excessive stress on the joints.

Hydrotherapy sessions are typically conducted in specialized pools or aquatic therapy centers, under the guidance of healthcare professionals or physical therapists. They can tailor exercises and techniques based on individual needs and conditions. However, hydrotherapy can also be practiced in natural bodies of water, as long as proper precautions and safety measures are followed.

If you're considering hydrotherapy as a part of your treatment plan, it's important to consult with your healthcare provider or a qualified aquatic therapist. They can assess your condition, recommend specific exercises, and provide guidance on the frequency and duration of hydrotherapy sessions based on your individual needs.

Overall, hydrotherapy can be a valuable therapeutic approach for joint relief, increased mobility, and overall well-being. Its benefits, combined with other treatment modalities, can contribute to an effective management plan for various joint conditions.

Exploring the Benefits of Hydrotherapy for Rheumatoid Arthritis

Hydrotherapy can offer several benefits for individuals with rheumatoid arthritis (RA). Here are some ways in which hydrotherapy can be beneficial for managing RA symptoms:

1. Pain Relief

Immersion in warm water during hydrotherapy sessions can provide pain relief for individuals with RA. The warmth helps relax muscles, reduces muscle spasms, and increases blood flow to the joints. This can alleviate pain and stiffness, promoting greater comfort and improved joint mobility.

2. Joint Mobility and Flexibility

The buoyancy of water in hydrotherapy reduces the impact on the joints, making movements easier and less painful. This allows individuals with RA to perform exercises and stretches that may be challenging on land. The gentle resistance provided by water also helps improve joint flexibility and range of motion.

3. Muscle Strength and Endurance

Hydrotherapy exercises in water offer a low-impact way to build and maintain muscle strength. The resistance provided by water helps strengthen the muscles surrounding the affected joints without putting excessive stress on them. Stronger muscles can provide better support to the joints and enhance overall joint stability.

4. Reduced Inflammation

Cold water hydrotherapy can be beneficial during RA flare-ups when joint inflammation is present. Cold water helps reduce inflammation, swelling, and pain in the affected joints. Alternating between warm and cold water can also have a soothing effect and help manage RA-related inflammation.

5. Relaxation and Stress Reduction

Hydrotherapy sessions can provide a relaxing and stress-reducing experience. The warmth of the water, gentle movements, and the overall calming environment can promote relaxation and alleviate stress. Stress reduction is important for individuals with RA as stress can worsen symptoms and contribute to disease flares.

6. Improved Sleep

Hydrotherapy can contribute to better sleep quality for individuals with RA. The relaxation and pain-relieving effects of hydrotherapy can help individuals experience more restful sleep, which is essential for managing RA symptoms and overall well-being.

It's important to note that hydrotherapy for RA should be done under the guidance of a healthcare professional, such as a physical therapist or hydrotherapist, who can develop a tailored treatment plan based on individual needs and limitations. They can provide specific exercises, monitor progress, and ensure safety during hydrotherapy sessions.

Before starting hydrotherapy or any new treatment, it's recommended to consult with your healthcare provider or rheumatologist to ensure it's suitable for your specific condition.

They can provide personalized guidance and determine if hydrotherapy should be incorporated into your overall RA management plan.

Water-Based Exercises: Enhancing Strength, Flexibility, and Balance

Water-based exercises are a highly effective way to enhance strength, flexibility, and balance while minimizing the impact on joints. These exercises, performed in water during hydrotherapy or aquatic therapy sessions, offer a range of benefits for individuals with various conditions or those seeking low-impact workouts.

Here's how water-based exercises can help improve strength, flexibility, and balance:

1. Resistance Training
Water provides natural resistance that challenges muscles throughout the body. Moving through water requires exertion, which strengthens muscles and promotes overall body strength. Water resistance can be adjusted by altering the speed and surface area of movement, making it suitable for individuals of different fitness levels.

2. Joint-Friendly
The buoyancy of water reduces the stress on joints, making it an ideal environment for exercise, especially for those with conditions like arthritis or joint pain. Water-based exercises allow for improved joint mobility and flexibility without subjecting the joints to excessive strain or impact. This enables individuals to perform movements that may be difficult or painful on land.

3. Full-Body Workout

Water-based exercises engage multiple muscle groups simultaneously, providing a comprehensive full-body workout. Movements such as water walking, swimming strokes, or aquatic aerobics involve the arms, legs, core, and even the resistance of water against the body. This helps improve overall muscle tone, endurance, and cardiovascular fitness.

4. Flexibility and Range of Motion

The water's buoyancy reduces the impact of gravity, allowing for increased joint range of motion and enhanced flexibility. Water-based exercises promote gentle stretching and elongation of muscles, improving flexibility and reducing muscle tightness. The warmth of the water during hydrotherapy can also aid in relaxing muscles and promoting flexibility.

5. Balance and Stability

Water-based exercises challenge balance and stability due to the constant shifting and resistance of water. Performing exercises in water requires core engagement and coordination, promoting better balance and proprioception. This is particularly beneficial for individuals at risk of falls or those with balance-related conditions.

6. Low-Impact Cardiovascular Conditioning

Water exercises can provide cardiovascular benefits without placing excessive stress on the joints. Activities such as water aerobics, water jogging, or swimming strokes can elevate the heart rate, improve cardiovascular fitness, and burn calories in a low-impact manner.

When engaging in water-based exercises, it's important to work with a qualified aquatic therapist or healthcare professional who can guide you through appropriate exercises and techniques. They can provide modifications, monitor your progress, and ensure safety during the sessions.

Whether you're participating in hydrotherapy or simply enjoying aquatic exercise for its benefits, water-based exercises offer a versatile and joint-friendly way to enhance strength, flexibility, and balance. Regular participation in these exercises can contribute to overall physical fitness, improved mobility, and increased well-being.

The Healing Power of Warm Water Pools: Reducing Joint Pressure and Promoting Relaxation

Warm water pools provide a therapeutic environment that can have a healing effect on the body, particularly for individuals with joint-related conditions or those seeking relaxation. The combination of warm water and buoyancy offers several benefits, including the reduction of joint pressure and the promotion of relaxation.

Here's how warm water pools can be beneficial:

1. Reduced Joint Pressure

The buoyancy of water reduces the effect of gravity on the body, providing a weightless sensation. This buoyancy helps alleviate the pressure on joints, allowing for greater freedom of movement with minimal stress. Immersion in a warm water pool can relieve joint pain and stiffness by supporting the body's weight and reducing the load on weight-bearing joints, such as the knees, hips, and spine.

2. Improved Joint Mobility

Warm water pools provide a gentle and supportive environment for joint movement. The warmth of the water helps relax muscles and increase blood flow to the joints, improving flexibility and range of motion. This can be particularly beneficial for individuals with conditions like arthritis or musculoskeletal disorders, as the warm water can help ease joint stiffness and enhance mobility.

3. Muscle Relaxation

The warm temperature of the water in a pool promotes muscle relaxation and can help reduce muscle tension. Warmth has a soothing effect on the muscles, relieving pain and promoting overall relaxation. This relaxation response can be beneficial for individuals with chronic pain or muscle tightness.

4. Circulation Enhancement

Warm water pools can improve blood circulation throughout the body. The warm temperature causes blood vessels to dilate, allowing for increased blood flow to muscles and joints. Enhanced circulation can aid in the delivery of oxygen and nutrients to tissues, while also facilitating the removal of waste products, promoting healing and tissue repair.

5. Stress Reduction and Relaxation

Immersion in a warm water pool has a calming and relaxing effect on the mind and body. The warm water, combined with the weightlessness and support provided by buoyancy, helps reduce stress and tension. It can promote relaxation, improve mood, and provide a sense of well-being. This can be particularly beneficial for individuals experiencing chronic pain or high levels of stress.

6. Safe Exercise Environment

Warm water pools offer a safe and supportive environment for exercise. The buoyancy and reduced joint pressure allow for low-impact movements and exercises that are gentle on the joints. Water-based exercises in a warm water pool can help improve strength, flexibility, and cardiovascular fitness without placing excessive stress on the body.

It's important to note that individuals with certain medical conditions, such as cardiovascular problems or infections, should consult with a healthcare professional before using warm water pools. Additionally, it's recommended to work with a qualified aquatic therapist or healthcare professional to receive guidance on appropriate exercises and techniques that suit your specific needs and limitations.

Overall, warm water pools provide a therapeutic and relaxing environment that can reduce joint pressure, promote muscle relaxation, enhance circulation, and improve overall well-being. Regular use of warm water pools, in combination with appropriate exercises and relaxation techniques, can contribute to better joint health and a sense of physical and mental rejuvenation.

Hydrotherapy as a Social and Emotional Support System

Hydrotherapy not only provides physical benefits but can also serve as a social and emotional support system. Participating in hydrotherapy sessions or engaging in water-based activities can offer opportunities for social interaction, emotional well-being, and a sense of community. Here's how hydrotherapy can serve as a social and emotional support system:

1. Group Environment

Hydrotherapy sessions often take place in group settings, allowing individuals to interact with others who may be experiencing similar health conditions or challenges. This group environment fosters a sense of belonging and creates opportunities for social connections. Sharing experiences, challenges, and successes with others can provide a supportive and empathetic network.

2. Peer Support

Engaging in hydrotherapy with peers can offer valuable emotional support. Interacting with individuals who are going through similar experiences can provide a sense of understanding, validation, and camaraderie. Sharing stories, strategies, and coping mechanisms can foster a sense of community and help individuals feel less isolated.

3. Encouragement and Motivation

In a hydrotherapy group, individuals often witness and celebrate each other's progress and achievements. This supportive atmosphere can be encouraging and motivating, inspiring individuals to continue their treatment journey and maintain a positive mindset. The shared determination and support from others can boost morale and help individuals overcome challenges.

4. Relaxation and Stress Reduction

Hydrotherapy's calming and soothing effects can contribute to emotional well-being and stress reduction. The warm water, gentle movements, and overall ambiance of a hydrotherapy session can help individuals relax, unwind, and temporarily escape from the stresses of daily life. This relaxation can promote emotional balance and mental clarity.

5. Increased Confidence and Self-Esteem

Engaging in hydrotherapy and witnessing personal progress can boost self-confidence and self-esteem. Overcoming physical challenges, improving mobility, and achieving personal goals in a supportive environment can enhance a person's sense of self-worth and empower them to take an active role in their own well-being.

6. Sense of Empowerment

Hydrotherapy empowers individuals by giving them a proactive role in managing their health. Participating in hydrotherapy exercises and adhering to a treatment plan can foster a sense of control and empowerment over one's own health journey. This sense of empowerment can positively impact emotional well-being and resilience.

It's important to note that while hydrotherapy can provide social and emotional support, the level of interaction and support may vary depending on the specific hydrotherapy program, group dynamics, and individual preferences. It's advisable to discuss any specific social or emotional needs with the healthcare professionals or therapists overseeing the hydrotherapy sessions to ensure that appropriate support is available.

In summary, hydrotherapy can serve as a social and emotional support system by providing opportunities for social interaction, peer support, encouragement, relaxation, and empowerment. The sense of community and emotional well-being derived from engaging in hydrotherapy can contribute to a more holistic approach to health and well-being.

Incorporating Hydrotherapy into Your Rheumatoid Arthritis Management Plan

Incorporating hydrotherapy into your rheumatoid arthritis (RA) management plan can provide numerous benefits for symptom relief, improved joint mobility, and overall well-being. Here are some steps to consider when integrating hydrotherapy into your RA management:

1. Consult with Your Healthcare Team

Before starting hydrotherapy or making any changes to your RA management plan, it's important to consult with your rheumatologist or healthcare team. They can evaluate your specific condition, assess any limitations or precautions, and provide guidance on incorporating hydrotherapy into your overall treatment strategy.

2. Seek a Qualified Hydrotherapy Professional

Look for a qualified hydrotherapist, aquatic therapist, or physical therapist experienced in working with individuals with RA or similar conditions. They can guide you through appropriate exercises, monitor your progress, and ensure your safety during hydrotherapy sessions.

3. Customize Your Hydrotherapy Program

Work with your hydrotherapist to create a customized hydrotherapy program that addresses your specific needs and goals. This may involve a combination of exercises, stretches, and relaxation techniques tailored to your abilities and limitations. Your program may also include specific focus areas such as joint flexibility, muscle strength, and pain management.

4. Start Slowly and Gradually Increase Intensity

Begin your hydrotherapy program at a pace that suits your comfort level and gradually increase the intensity and duration of exercises over time. This progressive approach allows your body to adapt and helps minimize the risk of overexertion or joint strain. Listen to your body and communicate any discomfort or concerns with your hydrotherapist.

5. Practice Consistently

Consistency is key for reaping the benefits of hydrotherapy. Aim for regular hydrotherapy sessions as part of your overall RA management plan. Your hydrotherapist can advise on an appropriate frequency, taking into account your specific needs and the availability of hydrotherapy facilities.

6. Combine Hydrotherapy with Other Treatments

Hydrotherapy can complement other RA treatments, such as medication, physical therapy, and lifestyle modifications. Integrating hydrotherapy into a comprehensive approach allows for a synergistic effect in managing your symptoms. Discuss with your healthcare team how hydrotherapy can be incorporated alongside other treatments to optimize your RA management plan.

7. Monitor and Evaluate Progress

Keep track of your progress throughout your hydrotherapy journey. Note any improvements in joint mobility, pain levels, and overall well-being. Regularly communicate with your hydrotherapist and healthcare team, providing updates on your experiences and any adjustments that may be needed.

8. Maintain a Healthy Lifestyle

In addition to hydrotherapy, maintain a healthy lifestyle by following a balanced diet, engaging in regular physical activity, managing stress, and getting enough restorative sleep. These lifestyle factors can further support your RA management and overall well-being.

Remember, hydrotherapy is just one component of your RA management plan. It's important to continue working closely with your healthcare team to ensure a comprehensive and individualized approach to managing your condition. They can provide ongoing support, monitor your progress, and make any necessary adjustments to your treatment plan.

Chapter 8

Tai Chi: Movement, Mindfulness, and Balance for Rheumatoid Arthritis

T'ai chi ch'üan, or simply "Tai chi," is a Chinese internal martial art that is practiced for meditation, health benefits, and self-defense training. It is often referred to as "shadowboxing". Tai Chi is a mind-body practice that combines gentle movements, deep breathing, and focused attention. It originated in ancient China and is often described as "meditation in motion." Tai Chi has gained popularity worldwide for its numerous health benefits, including its potential benefits for individuals with rheumatoid arthritis (RA).

Rheumatoid arthritis is a chronic autoimmune condition characterized by inflammation and pain in the joints. It can lead to reduced mobility, balance problems, and overall decreased quality of life. While there is no cure for RA, there are various management strategies, and incorporating Tai Chi into the routine may offer several advantages.

1. Gentle Movements

Tai Chi consists of slow, flowing movements that help improve joint flexibility, strength, and range of motion without putting excessive stress on the joints. The gentle nature of the practice makes it suitable for individuals with RA, as it can help alleviate stiffness and reduce pain.

2. Mindfulness and Relaxation

Tai Chi emphasizes mindful awareness and relaxation. By focusing on the present moment and the sensations in the body, individuals with RA can develop a better understanding of their pain and learn to manage it more effectively. The practice can also reduce stress and anxiety, which are common in individuals with chronic conditions like RA.

3. Balance and Coordination

RA can affect balance and increase the risk of falls. Tai Chi incorporates weight shifting, coordinated movements, and postural control, which can help improve balance and stability. Regular practice may enhance muscle strength and proprioception, reducing the likelihood of falls and related injuries.

4. Low-Impact Exercise

Tai Chi is a low-impact exercise that puts minimal stress on the joints. This makes it a suitable option for individuals with RA who may have joint damage or pain. Unlike high-impact activities like running or jumping, Tai Chi provides a gentle form of exercise that can be adapted to individual abilities.

When considering Tai Chi for managing rheumatoid arthritis, it is important to consult with a healthcare professional or a qualified Tai Chi instructor who has experience working with individuals with RA. They can provide guidance on modifications to accommodate specific needs and limitations. Additionally, it is crucial to listen to your body, start slowly, and gradually increase the intensity and duration of the practice as tolerated.

Overall, Tai Chi can be a valuable addition to a comprehensive management plan for rheumatoid arthritis. Its combination of gentle movements, mindfulness, and balance training can promote physical and emotional well-being, improve joint function, and enhance overall quality of life for individuals living with RA.

Understanding the Foundations of Tai Chi: Balance, Flow, and Mindfulness

The foundations of Tai Chi revolve around three key elements: balance, flow, and mindfulness. These principles form the core of the practice and contribute to its holistic benefits for both physical and mental well-being.

1. Balance

Balance is fundamental in Tai Chi. It refers to both physical balance and the concept of finding balance in life. In terms of physical balance, Tai Chi movements often involve shifting weight from one leg to another, maintaining a stable center of gravity, and promoting an upright posture. This focus on balance can help improve stability, coordination, and reduce the risk of falls. It also extends to finding a balance between different aspects of life, such as work and leisure, rest and activity, and emotional well-being.

2. Flow

Flow refers to the continuous, smooth, and connected movements in Tai Chi. Practitioners strive for a seamless transition between different postures and transitions. Flowing movements help cultivate a sense of grace, ease, and harmony in the body. By emphasizing the flow of energy, or "qi," throughout the body, Tai

Chi aims to improve circulation, promote relaxation, and enhance the body's natural healing abilities. Flowing movements also help to release tension, improve flexibility, and increase body awareness.

3. Mindfulness

Mindfulness is a central component of Tai Chi practice. It involves cultivating a focused awareness of the present moment, without judgment or distraction. In Tai Chi, practitioners aim to bring their attention to the sensations in their body, their breath, and the movements they are performing. By being fully present in the practice, individuals can deepen their mind-body connection, improve concentration, and reduce stress. Mindfulness in Tai Chi extends beyond the practice itself and can be applied to daily life, promoting a more mindful and balanced approach to various situations.

Combining these three foundations, Tai Chi offers a unique integration of physical movement, mental focus, and breath control. The practice encourages individuals to cultivate a state of calmness, centeredness, and self-awareness. Through regular practice, Tai Chi can promote physical fitness, improve flexibility and balance, enhance mental clarity and emotional well-being, and foster a sense of overall harmony and well-being.

It's important to note that learning Tai Chi is best done under the guidance of a qualified instructor who can provide proper instruction, correct form, and guidance tailored to individual needs and abilities.

The Physical and Mental Benefits of Tai Chi for Rheumatoid Arthritis

Tai Chi offers several physical and mental benefits for individuals with rheumatoid arthritis (RA). Here are some of the potential advantages:

1. Joint Health and Flexibility

The gentle, flowing movements of Tai Chi can help improve joint flexibility, range of motion, and lubrication. Regular practice can reduce stiffness in the joints affected by RA, promoting better mobility and joint health.

2. Muscle Strength and Endurance

Tai Chi involves controlled movements that engage various muscle groups. Through continuous practice, it can help strengthen muscles, particularly those surrounding the affected joints. Stronger muscles provide better support to the joints, potentially reducing pain and improving overall endurance.

3. Balance and Fall Prevention

Individuals with RA may experience balance problems, which can increase the risk of falls. Tai Chi emphasizes weight shifting, coordination, and postural control, all of which can improve balance and stability. Enhanced balance reduces the likelihood of falls and related injuries.

4. Pain Management

Tai Chi's slow, gentle movements and mindfulness-based approach can help individuals with RA manage pain. By focusing on the present moment and the sensations in the body, Tai Chi cultivates a better understanding of pain and enables individuals to develop techniques for coping with discomfort.

5. Stress Reduction and Emotional Well-being

Chronic conditions like RA can take a toll on mental and emotional health. Tai Chi incorporates mindfulness and relaxation techniques, helping to reduce stress, anxiety, and depression. It promotes a sense of calmness, inner peace, and emotional well-being.

6. Improved Sleep

Sleep disturbances are common in individuals with RA, and Tai Chi has been shown to improve sleep quality. The relaxation techniques and mindful focus in Tai Chi can promote a deeper and more restful sleep, leading to better overall health and vitality.

7. Enhanced Quality of Life

The combination of physical benefits, pain management, stress reduction, and improved emotional well-being can greatly enhance the overall quality of life for individuals with RA. Tai Chi offers a holistic approach that addresses both the physical and mental aspects of living with a chronic condition.

It is worth noting that while Tai Chi can provide numerous benefits for individuals with RA, it should not replace medical treatment or other interventions recommended by healthcare professionals. It is important to consult with a healthcare provider or a qualified Tai Chi instructor who can offer guidance tailored to individual needs and limitations. They can help adapt the practice to suit individual abilities and ensure a safe and effective approach.

Tailoring Tai Chi for Joint Health and Mobility Enhancement

Tailoring Tai Chi for joint health and mobility enhancement is a great way to leverage the benefits of this ancient Chinese martial art and mind-body practice. Tai Chi is known for its slow, flowing movements, which can be adapted and modified to address specific joint issues and improve overall mobility. Here are some suggestions on how to tailor Tai Chi for joint health and mobility enhancement:

1. Seek guidance from a qualified instructor

Working with a knowledgeable Tai Chi instructor is essential, especially when tailoring the practice for joint health. They can provide guidance on appropriate modifications and help you understand the principles behind the movements.

2. Warm-up exercises

Begin your Tai Chi practice with warm-up exercises specifically designed to lubricate the joints and increase blood flow. Gentle joint rotations, ankle pumps, and wrist circles can be incorporated to prepare your body for the practice.

3. Modify movements for joint comfort

If you have joint limitations or specific areas of concern, make modifications to Tai Chi movements to suit your needs. For example, if you have knee issues, you can slightly bend your knees instead of performing deep knee bends. Experiment with different variations that alleviate joint stress while still maintaining the essence of the movement.

4. Focus on gentle stretching

Tai Chi provides an opportunity for gentle stretching, which can improve joint flexibility. Emphasize movements that involve stretching the joints, such as "Grasp the Sparrow's Tail" or "White Crane Spreads Its Wings." Pay attention to your body's feedback and avoid overstretching or pushing beyond your limits.

5. Slow and controlled movements

Tai Chi is known for its slow and deliberate movements, which allow for increased body awareness and control. By moving slowly and mindfully, you can reduce joint impact while maintaining a focus on joint alignment and stability.

6. Incorporate balance exercises

Balance is closely linked to joint health and mobility. Integrate balance exercises into your Tai Chi practice, such as standing on one leg or performing weight shifts. These exercises challenge the joints and improve overall stability.

7. Mind-body connection

Tai Chi is not just about physical movements but also about cultivating a strong mind-body connection. Use this aspect to your advantage by directing your attention to the joints during the practice. Visualize the movements as promoting joint health and mobility, and cultivate a sense of relaxation and mindfulness.

8. Practice regularly

Consistency is key when it comes to reaping the benefits of Tai Chi for joint health and mobility. Aim for regular practice sessions, even if they are shorter in duration. Gradually increase the practice duration as your body becomes more accustomed to the movements.

Remember to listen to your body and consult with a healthcare professional if you have any underlying medical conditions or concerns. Tai Chi can be a valuable tool for joint health and mobility enhancement when tailored to suit your individual needs.

Incorporating Tai Chi into Your Daily Routine: Practicing at Home or Joining a Class

Incorporating Tai Chi into your daily routine can bring numerous benefits to your overall well-being. Whether you choose to practice at home or join a class, here are some considerations to help you get started:

Practicing at Home:

1. **Find a suitable space:** Look for a quiet and well-ventilated area in your home where you can practice Tai Chi without distractions. Make sure you have enough space to move around comfortably, with no furniture or obstacles in your way.

2. **Set a regular schedule:** Establish a consistent practice schedule that works for you. Consistency is key to reaping the benefits of Tai Chi. Decide on the best time of day for your practice, whether it's morning, afternoon, or evening, and allocate a specific duration for your sessions.

3. **Warm-up exercises:** Begin your home practice with gentle warm-up exercises to prepare your body for Tai Chi. Incorporate joint rotations, stretches, and deep breathing exercises to loosen up your muscles and enhance flexibility.

4. **Follow a structured routine:** If you're new to Tai Chi or prefer guidance, consider using instructional videos, books, or online resources that provide structured routines or sequences. Start with beginner-level material and gradually progress as you become more comfortable with the movements.

5. **Pay attention to form and technique:** Proper form is crucial in Tai Chi. Focus on maintaining correct posture, alignment, and body mechanics as you perform the movements. Remember to move slowly, with fluidity and control, while engaging your core and maintaining relaxed and balanced movements.

6. **Mind-body connection:** Tai Chi is a mind-body practice that emphasizes mindfulness and relaxation. Cultivate a sense of calmness and focus during your practice. Pay attention to your breath, the sensations in your body, and the meditative aspects of the movements.

Joining a Class:

1. **Find a qualified instructor:** Look for Tai Chi classes or workshops in your local community or online. Seek instructors who have experience and certification in teaching Tai Chi. They can guide you through proper techniques and provide personalized feedback.

2. **Determine the class format:** Tai Chi classes can vary in their structure and focus. Some classes may emphasize the martial aspects, while others may prioritize health and relaxation. Choose a class that aligns with your goals and interests.

3. **Consider the class level:** Classes are typically offered at different levels, such as beginner, intermediate, and

advanced. Assess your experience and skill level to select a class that suits your needs. Starting with a beginner-level class allows you to build a strong foundation.

4. **Attend regularly:** Commit to attending classes regularly to experience the full benefits of Tai Chi. Consistent practice under the guidance of an instructor helps refine your technique, deepen your understanding, and foster a supportive learning environment.

5. **Practice outside of class:** Supplement your class attendance with home practice. Practicing Tai Chi at home allows you to reinforce what you've learned in class and develop a deeper connection with the movements. Your instructor can provide guidance on how to structure your home practice sessions.

Remember to listen to your body, take breaks as needed, and progress at your own pace. Whether you choose to practice at home or join a class, Tai Chi can become a fulfilling and transformative part of your daily routine.

References

https://en.m.wikipedia.org/wiki/Massage

https://en.m.wikipedia.org/wiki/Tai_chi

https://www.arthritis.org/health-wellness/treatment/complementary-therapies/natural-therapies/meditation-benefits-for-people-with-arthritis

https://www.everydayhealth.com/rheumatoid-arthritis/living-with/can-mindfulness-meditation-ease-arthritis-pain/

https://www.hindawi.com/journals/ecam/2018/8596918/

https://www.mayoclinic.org/tests-procedures/acupuncture/about/pac-20392763#

https://www.medicalnewstoday.com/articles/156488#uses

https://www.ncbi.nlm.nih.gov/books/NBK532287/

https://www.ncbi.nlm.nih.gov/pmc/articles/PMC5925010/

https://www.nccih.nih.gov/health/acupuncture-what-you-need-to-know

https://www.tikvahlake.com/blog/the-best-mind-body-techniques-for-managing-stress/

https://www.versusarthritis.org/news/2022/february/meditation-and-mindfulness-and-how-it-might-help-you/

www.ingramcontent.com/pod-product-compliance
Lightning Source LLC
Chambersburg PA
CBHW070126260726
48658CB00001B/279